A Blending of American and Chinese Theory

The Nuts, Bolts & Greens of a Healthy Back

by
Dr. Marcia Schmidt

PERQ Publications®

© 1999 by Dr. Marcia Schmidt

Published by PERQ Publications®
a division of Professional Resources & Communications, Inc.
509 West Main Street
Barrington, IL 60010
800/236-4303
www.prcinc.net/perq.htm

Printed in the United States of America

ISBN: 1-880439-06-9

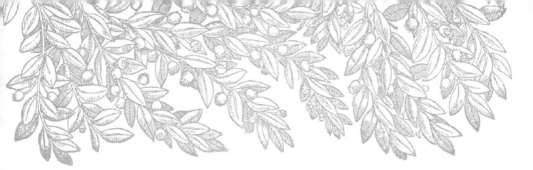

Dedication

To Joan who put a tape recorder in my hand.

To Bruce who guided me to computer literacy.

And mostly to Becky, the brilliant light of my life who was the first to imagine this book.

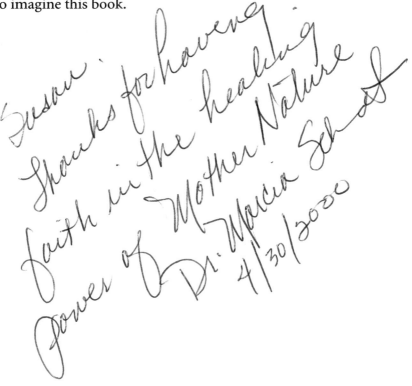

Susan,
Thanks for having
faith in the healing
power of Mother Nature
Dr. Marcia Schnedler
4/30/2000

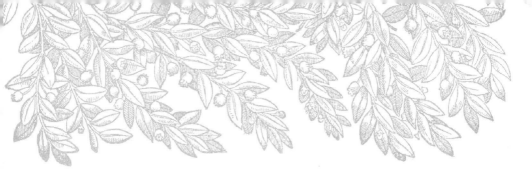

Contents

About This Book's Structure ....**vii**

Foreword ....**ix**

Preface ....**xi**

Chapter 1
Calcium and Minerals and Their Importance **1**

Chapter 2
Muscle, Bone, and Naprapathy..**11**

Chapter 3
Lower Back and "Lower" **33**

Chapter 4
Neck Care..**55**

Chapter 5
Help for Headaches...**69**

Chapter 6
Easing Nerves, Depression, and Stress **85**

Chapter 7
Recharging Your Batteries...**111**

Chapter 8
Dr. Schmidt's Favorite Compresses **129**

Chapter 9
Favorite Chinese Remedies...**135**

Chapter 10
Naprapathic History **147**

Afterword **163**
Contacts **165**
Index **171**

About This Book's Structure

This book is arranged just as if you had walked into my office for the first time. Since most of you arrive with muscular and skeletal problems, I begin with a discussion of the proper nutrition for these structures, how to get those nutrients where we want them, and what to expect from the cleansing action of the first treatment. My evaluation of your area of complaint corresponds with the chapters on low back, neck, and headache. Here the reader will learn how to touch, evaluate for themselves, and begin their own road to recovery.

The chapters containing less tangible problems, such as nerves, stress, tension, and depression, follow next. Once you relax on my treatment table, our conversation inevitably leads to the every day concerns of your life that create your whole health picture. As we unravel the complexities of this picture, we can draw from a pharmacopoeia of natural remedies, herbal compresses, ancient oriental liniments, exercises, wild foods, and the most powerful tool you possess—your mind—which make up the end of the book.

The chapter called Recharging Your Batteries contains Dr. Schmidt's favorite power foods, affirmations and breathing techniques, and a trip to a natural hot spring that can help you reclaim that vital energy that you had as a child.

The final chapter is the history of naprapathy from 1899: its origination from chiropractic beginnings, years of political and licenser uncertainty, and the road of compromise I had to take toward medical freedom.

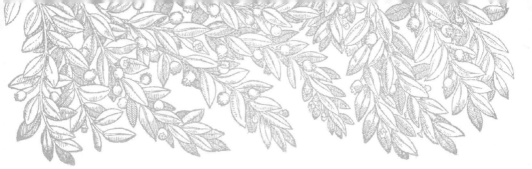

Foreword

By Dr. Rosita Arvigo, D.N.

As a fellow doctor of naprapathy, I know that a book like this is long overdue and will no doubt find an enthusiastic audience. At a time when natural treatments for human ailments are experiencing a great following, it is essential that proper education be available to the public. Many would prefer to try natural therapies before opting for more invasive treatments, but do not know how to start or where to go for help. This book fills that need nicely. It is written by a person of great experience in the field and whose feet are planted firmly on the ground. Doctor Schmidt gives some good and basic common sense advice on treating backaches, headaches, and muscle spasms with naprapathic treatments and a host of simple home remedies which have been tried and shown to be true throughout the ages. Some of them I know well and use in my own family practice with the same good results over the past thirty years.

It is particularly interesting to see how the author has woven traditional Chinese Medicine and modern body work into a coherent and sensible tapestry. The case studies and personal experiences she shares give the book a homey feeling which should appeal to a large number of people within and without the healing professions.

Dr. Schmidt and I agree that a physician must always get to the cause of the physical ailment and that treating the symptoms without removing the underlying cause leads to frustration and disappointment in both practitioner and patient. Helping people to understand how they got on a road that led to illness and then showing them the way back out of darkness into light is a great gift, indeed. There is often no simple or single cause, especially for musculoskeletal ailments, but it is the domain of the natural practitioner to uncover the details of the multiple causation for the patient and then point the way to full recovery with relief of symptoms. Along the road to recovery the patient needs assistance with diet, exercise, supplements, herbs, meditation, relaxation, and naprapathic treatments. Addressing the needs of the body, mind, and soul in healing is now the bridge that will lead us into the next millennium: a time, we hope, when allopathic doctors and natural healers will find common ground in order to alleviate the suffering of all humankind.

I applaud the publication of this book and counsel the reader to put these bits of wisdom and experience to use in everyday life, because they come from one who is blessed with the ability to make what is confusing simple and what is intimidating approachable.

Dr. Arvigo is one of the world's leading Ethnobotanical authorities of the Rainforest at Belize, Central America, and Director of the Belize Ethnobotany Project through the Ix Chel Tropical Research Foundation, the New York Botanical Garden Institute of Economic Botany, along with the National Cancer Institutes' sponsored Collection Program.

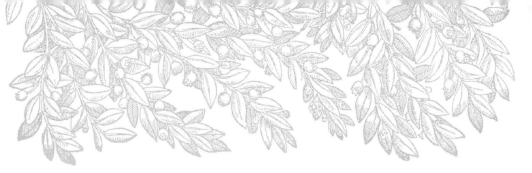

Preface

This book is not a list of vitamins and herbs and the 101 illnesses they will cure. Rather, it is a compassionate look into the lives of a few of my patients as they attempt to find health using Mother Nature's tools. Interspersed among the nuts, bolts, and greens of minerals, castor oil packs, and naprapathic and massage techniques are the real stories of the complicated nature of people's lives—the dis-ease of their backs and shoulders; sciatic nerve pains; headaches; carpal tunnel syndrome; depression; and simple aches and strains—all those problems that represent a fall from the perfect balance available to us all when we pattern our lives after Mother Nature's examples.

This book tells the story of how an ancient Chinese healer came into my life to show me that the simplicity of nature is the pervading wisdom one should always use when evaluating this fall from perfect balance. Most Western alternative practitioners throw a dart at the chart of ten recommended herbs for any disease. For instance, echinacea, goldenseal, chamomile, or astragalus are all natural antibiotics—just pick one when a patient walks in with a cold. The oriental system of evaluating and administering herbs has much more depth. The strengths and weakness of organs such as the lungs, liver, heart, and kidneys are considered and assessed in seconds, without expensive hospital procedures or a giant hole in your savings account. Factors such as heat or cold in diet and body structure influence therapy plans. When such vital information is combined with the naprapath's ability to get the blood carrying these medicinal herbs to the area of weakness, you get a livable solution to your pain—a solution that does not require visiting a chiropractor's office once a week for the rest of your life.

You will learn that pain is your body's alarm system, and that shutting it off may be the worst thing you can do. This ancient and profoundly wise shell that we walk around in sends signals, sometimes loudly and sometimes painfully, when its natural balance is disturbed. Learning to listen to these signals and becoming one with your body is one of the most important messages this book has to offer.

You won't find any silver bullets here—no cure-all-your-symptoms pill that your MD can give you to go on being "normal." Nonetheless, this book is not technical. There are only a handful of reasons that may contribute to your back going out, and the simple knowledge you gain from this book should help you detect them. With that knowledge, and such easily available remedies as apple cider vinegar, and maybe a few dandelions, you can take responsibility for your own health.

In 1981, I was a woodworker employed in my father's business, refinishing fine antiques and making furniture and signs. It was at this time that Gordon Schurzer, a high school friend, told me that he was studying to be a naprapath. I had never heard of a naprapath (pronounced *NAP-pra-path)* or the profession of naprapathy (pronounced *na-PRA-pa-thee*). I didn't know that naprapathy is a system of treatment that utilizes manipulation of muscles, ligaments, and tendons, in conjunction with dietary measures, to facilitate the wonderful recuperative and regenerative powers of the body. I couldn't even pronounce it. Yet, when he said he needed a willing victim to practice on, I was first in line to try anything that felt like a great massage while making me healthier at the same time.

Dr. Gordon would come to my apartment on Sunday nights after long hours of studying and classes. After eating anything in the refrigerator that didn't move, we would throw a blanket on the front room floor, and I would give him great back, shoulder, and neck massages. He would then show me some of the techniques he'd learned that week in school, assuring me I would be a great naprapath. He said I had the hands for it. I never guessed that rubbing my mother's shoulders every night after dinner would lead me to my life's passion and my gift to mankind. Today, my hands are tremendously sensitive. I can instantly feel tightness, obstructions in energy, and even lack of proper circulation.

Dr. Gordon had me thoroughly convinced that this was my calling, until he related his accounts of cadaver class. The gory details of dissecting human body parts kept me from pursuing naprapathy for over a year! However, a tiny whisper in my soul assured me that I would surprise myself at what I would accomplish. A healing system that encouraged a drugless path to greater health and vitality, using your own hands as your tools, set my soul on fire.

The Chicago National College of Naprapathy was a roller-coaster ride in a tunnel whose only light was graduation day off in the distance. Working days, taking courses in the evenings, studying for long hours, and attending cadaver classes on Saturdays turned me into one sick girl. The long hours, continual stress, and poor eating habits taxed my immune system. My body was covered with red, swollen, itchy skin. It was ironic that my own health began to deteriorate right when I started studying for a medical career. Before I'd gotten my professional career off the ground, *I* was the one needing the most help from it. I searched for normalcy among herbs, vitamins, macrobiotic foods, colonics, and the gentle manipulation therapy of naprapathy. Then I met Dr. Pak Lau. Dr. Gordon had told me that Dr. Lau and his daughter, Dr. Lisa Lau, had lectured on the principles of traditional Chinese medicine in Chicago's Chinatown. Dr. Lau does not speak English, so his daughter, also a traditional Oriental Medical Doctor (OMD), interprets for him.

Dr. Lau is small and slightly balding, with marvelously smooth skin. In fact, my patients who've met him joke that he's magically preserved, never having changed over the 15 years I've known him. With his long delicate fingers, he can take three superficial and three deep pulses from the radial artery on each of your wrists. These pulses, which I describe as being similar to the electrical current that flows through a house, supply energy to the body's twelve organ systems. They start at the feet, work up to the head, down the arms, and down the back of the body to the feet, as they convey vibrating energy, electrons, protons, neutrons, or chi, the essence of life. Without an X-ray, CAT scan, or MRI, Dr. Lau can discern what organs are weak, how long they have been that way, and which one began the deficiency. He can tell what ailments you were born with and what you developed as a result of your living patterns. He is also an herbalist par excellence.

His office is part Chinese grocery, part Chinese pharmacy, and part video rental store. In the back, he has a waiting area and a tiny 8' x 10' office. Through the partition that separates the crowded waiting area from this tiny room are patients of every nationality, waiting to get Dr. Lau's advice concerning their health problems.

His tiny office is crowded with his desk, a chair for his daughter the interpreter, and two chairs for patients. One wall is lined with manila folders jammed with precious herbal recipes. From behind his desk, a large brightly-painted watercolor of an enormous goldfish (a symbol of great luck), in a traditional Chinese gold frame, overlooks the whole scene. There are portraits of grand-children with wonderfully warm smiles, being hugged or hugging someone. On Dr. Lau's desks sits a ceramic teapot, steeping tea with a strange aroma unfamiliar to my American nostrils. The wall behind the desk overflows with boxes. Some are filled with Chinese cough syrups and ginseng, queen-bee pollen and mush-rooms. Many others are filled with remedies whose uses I could only imagine. There is barely room to move.

Dr. Lisa calmly translated as I told my tale of school, stress and unexplained rashes. Dr. Lau's only English came when, with a large flashlight in hand, he demanded to see my tongue. I understood nothing of the solemn look on his face and the nod of his head. But since then, I have come to know that this is standard procedure. An appraisal of the tongue can provide a quick diagnosis of a patient's overall health. A rosy pink color indicates a

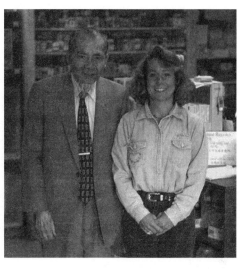

Dr. Pak Lau and myself

healthy system. A white tongue might indicate the body's accumulation of mucus and the need for cleansing. And yellow suggests a body that is not excreting toxins and wastes, meaning the colon needs cleansing.

After Dr. Lau took my pulses, he examined my eyes and face. Then questions like, "Eat good?" "Sleep good?" "Pee good?" and "Poop good?" were addressed. After great contemplation, he began writing on a plain piece of white paper. My Western eyes could only stare in wonder as he "drew" three vertical columns of an ancient herbal formula,

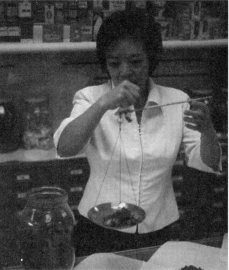

Dr. Lisa Lau, measuring herbs with an authentic chinese balance scale

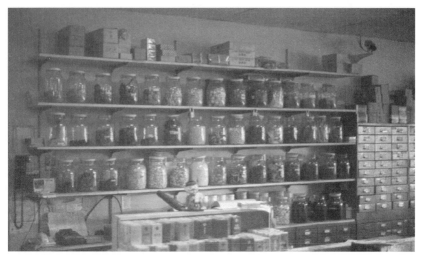

Dr. Lau's inventory of remedies

thousands of years old, in Chinese pictographs composed of flowing black strokes and slashes.

Dr. Lisa took my prescription to the front of the shop where the walls held hundreds of drawers filled with roots, stems, leaves, barks, dried squashed black things (even large dried bugs), and the skeletal remains of tiny seahorses. She carefully measured and weighed ten different herbs using a hand-held balance scale, and

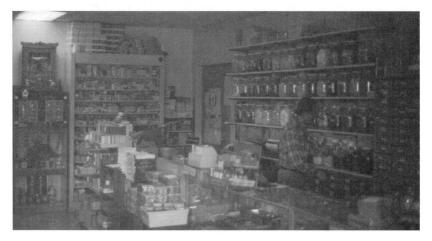

The inside of Dr. Lau's Store, and the vast number of remedies

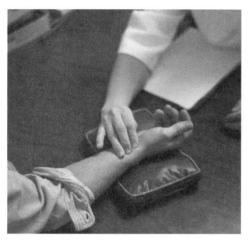

Dr. Lisa Lau, taking my pulse

placed them in the center of an eight-inch square of paper, securing it with a rubber band. I was given three packages containing the same herbal combination (this equaled about one week's worth of tea), and a little container of cream marked "no. 2." Under normal circumstances, I would have been sent home to brew my sacred concoction, but I was one of those rare patients who needed acupuncture. Apparently, some normal energy flow was stuck, causing the persistent rash that covered me from head to toe.

Dr. Lau pulled out his long silver acupuncture needles, carefully washed each insertion area with alcohol and painlessly applied

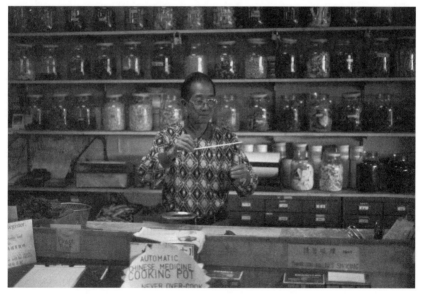

Dr. Lau's assistant weighing a presciption of herbs

needles to my face, forearms, belly and hands. He did not say a word, but busily rechecked each needle after insertion, poking them here, twisting them there—I was bewildered at the lack of pain and discomfort. Finally, he grabbed a stalk of dried herbs tied together with a heavy string and set it afire. As the smoke rose and intertwined itself around the needles, it delivered the additional energy that the burning herbs had to offer. I was amazed and uncomprehending. It was like entering a Third-World country in which I was a mere visitor, hoping that this strange path would lead to better health.

The needles inserted into my hands and arms left my thumbs with a vague lifelessness. But somehow, I managed to drive home without using them. Within hours, however, my thumb control returned and at the same time, I noticed the rash on my arms changing. After four days of drinking Dr. Lau's herbal concoction, the rash and itching were much better.

Over the years, I have sent patients to Dr. Lau who were appalled by his apparent lack of concern for American standards of cleanliness. I am saddened for these folks, who can't get beyond the clutter and the unusual setting to see an ancient medical system light years ahead of its time. This is a system that uses herbs that vibrate with our own body's frequency, resonate to healthy organs, and raise our level of health using the principles of Nature—wind, water, wood, air, fire, and cold—that Nature herself created. Many years ago, the Chinese observed these principles, which have remained unchanged since the beginning of time, and applied them to their daily lives and their system of healing. Mother Nature's gift is her simplicity.

Chapter 1

Calcium and Minerals and Their Importance

The last time you thought of the word "calcium," I'll bet you pictured a great, big white mustache on top of a familiar smile looking out from a magazine or a roadside sign. Those billboard celebrities comfort you with the assurance that you will always have strong bones and teeth when you drink milk. But guess what? Calcium is not only important for bones and teeth, it is extremely important for smooth muscle action. You may be horrified to find out that seventy percent of the calcium from a glass of milk is *not* absorbable,[1] and if you later choose a can of soda with a hamburger, you are stealing not only what little calcium the milk had to offer, but also calcium from your muscle and bone reserves. This results in muscle spasms, whether they are in your back, neck, jaw, or uterus, and if calcium depletion goes on long enough, it can cause osteoporosis. This book is about muscles, and how and why they need minerals—chiefly calcium and magnesium.

Awakening in the morning, Tom opened his eyes, almost forgetting his pain. Lying still, he felt all right, but that first move—his attempt to shift positions—frightened him. Silently, he did a mental assessment of yesterday's pain and stiffness.

Last weekend the 38-year-old Tom had played softball both Saturday and Sunday, but that was nothing new. Throughout each summer since he was in his early 20s, he played the game twice a week. Last Sunday, the temperature had been in the 90s (it was the middle of July,) and he had drunk soda pop all afternoon to keep cool. By late Monday afternoon, he began to get stiff. By noon on Tuesday, he was so stiff in his lower back and in the muscles of his buttocks that he tried not to bend over too far. By Wednesday, he couldn't even bend forward to answer the phone on his desk. The stiffness increased and pain accompanied any bending. A cough, sneeze, or (heaven forbid) a laugh brought tears to Tom's eyes from the sudden rush of unexpected pain.

That was Tom's story as he entered my office Wednesday evening. Something had to be done. He couldn't work, he couldn't drive, and standing up from a sitting position was almost impossible. How could a slim, active man, who was an occasional weight lifter and an enthusiastic softball player, fall apart like this?

Unraveling the how and why of Tom's back problems requires understanding both the muscular and skeletal systems of the body, and also understanding Tom. How much muscle power is he using? Is he ingesting the proper nutrients to use those muscles? Is anything competing with his muscles for those precious nutrients? What happens to his bones if the muscles are starved for the proper nutrition? How does Tom's job, and the duties he performs at that job, affect his back? How does his attitude about himself create his own health picture?

As an electrical engineer for a large electrical company, Tom spent most of his time walking around job sites, evaluating work in progress and determining what needed to be done next. Because these responsibilities required him to walk, climb, and drive quite a bit, he had on occasion experienced stiffness in his shoulders and lower back, but nothing this devastating. Moreover, he was certain that he had not fallen nor had any accident that would lead me to suspect a fracture in his spine or hips.

After more questioning, I also discovered that Tom considered himself to be a "meat and potatoes" guy. He ate few vegetables, but would take a multiple vitamin occasionally—usually at breakfast with one of the several cups of coffee he drank each day.

The Muscular-Skeletal System and Calcium

The muscular and skeletal systems are intertwined, so that a problem with one can create a problem with the other. Therefore, I would never assume that Tom's devastating pain originated only in his muscles or only in his bones.

You Are What You Eat, so Pack in the Minerals

To understand how our bodies lose their natural harmony, we need to open our eyes to Mother Earth. When we apply her patterns to our everyday lifestyles, we may reduce inflammation to muscles, bones, and nerves. We need to walk through Mother Nature's garden and choose her healing green medicinal herbs and vegetables in order to cool inflammation and promote circulation to irritated tissues, whether they involve muscle or bone. We must examine the peaceful harmony that pervades the entire universe and understand that we are what we think, do, and eat. We have the power to create the harmony we strive for, and also create the disharmony that can knock us to our knees when our lower back "goes out."

Eighty percent of the people I see have lost their perfect skeletal alignment because of an imbalance in their nutritional intake. Deficiencies in our diets can often affect soft tissues, creating muscular spasms, which in turn pull on the bones. Heavy proteins, such as beef, pork, lamb, and carbonated beverages (regular, diet, caffeinated or caffeine-free soda pop) are real culprits.[2]

The high level of phosphorous they contain can make our back muscles stiff as boards.[3]

Calcium is one of the body's major minerals. Phosphorous is essential to help our bodies *absorb* the calcium, while magnesium and vitamin D are essential for its proper *utilization*. But excess phosphorous can cause problems. Muscles have a sliding, gate-like mechanism that allows muscle fibers to expand and contract. A balance of calcium and magnesium allows muscle to contract and expand effectively. However, an *excess* of phosphorous from beef and soda pop obstructs this process.[4] As these large levels of phosphorus enter the digestive tract, alarm systems fire off warnings that the pH is going to turn too acidic for good health. Our precious calcium reserves surround the dangerous phosphorus and turn the pH back toward an alkaline range. One molecule of phosphorous binds with fifteen molecules of calcium. As this combination is carried through the bloodstream and eventually through the kidneys, it is sorted out as an undesirable or low threshold. As a result, the kidneys excrete precious calcium from the body as a protective mechanism to eliminate excess phosphorus. Most Americans consume two to three times the necessary daily requirements for protein, which results in inadequate calcium reserves.

While magnesium relaxes muscle tissue, calcium helps it contract, and so one might expect that a lack of calcium would cause the muscle to be limp or flaccid. Instead, the opposite occurs—the muscle contracts, binds, and refuses to let go. The calcium needed to prevent these muscle spasms passes out of the body through the kidneys, attached to phosphorous we don't need. I call this "the-baby-being-thrown-out-with-the-bath-water syndrome." This condition causes the stiffness we feel as we awake each morning. It is responsible for the tension in our necks and shoulders we describe as "an achiness" that won't let us turn our heads. And it results in the pain that builds throughout the day after we've bent down to pick up a single piece of paper and heard that "pop!" as our backs go out.

Further effects of this calcium dumping are seen when our muscles say, "Oh no, Mr. Phosphorous! I refuse to give you any more calcium. Go find your calcium from the bone reserves." Of course, when phosphorous siphons off calcium from the bones, the bones lose their inner matrix—their inner mineral makeup. This problem, called osteoporosis or bone thinning, is rampant in our wealthy population of meat eaters and soda pop drinkers.

Those of you reading casually *must* stop and pay attention. I have treated ailing backs for 12 years, and more than half of the people who could barely move because of their back pain recovered 100 percent by giving up carbonated beverages and limiting their intake of heavy proteins! Patients who occasionally let a piece of meat slide its way on to their plates must double their intake of calcium the same day (or even two days) after eating the meat. I don't want to sound like a broken record, or should I say CD, but I've seen more than one patient, still in pain after the best medical care at the Mayo Clinic, return to normal health by eliminating carbonated beverages and adding calcium in the form of green leafy vegetables or an herbal calcium supplement.

Sources for Calcium—Greens, Cooked or Raw, You Need Both
Calcium is the largest mineral in our bodies and requires vitamins A, C, D, and dietary magnesium and phosphorous to be properly absorbed. "Whoa!" you say. "Life is way too busy to have to open this bottle of vitamin A and that bottle of vitamin D, let alone magnesium, phosphorous, and vitamin C." The good news is—green foods have them all, plus chlorophyll. Chlorophyll is a valuable blood purifier that cools inflammation and rejuvenates naturally.

The best bio-available calcium, or the calcium most easily recognized and most efficiently absorbed, is *not* found in milk but in dark-green leafy foods. Seventy percent of the calcium found in dairy never makes it through the walls of the intestine and is simply excreted in the feces.[5] Milk is very good for little cows but we are human beings[6]. Generally, I don't recommend dairy products at all because of their potential to coat the colon walls with mucus.

SOURCES OF CALCIUM   *100-mg. (31/2 ounce) edible portions*

Food	Calcium in Milligrams (mg.)
Hijiki	1,400
Wakame	1,300
Kelp	1,099
Kombu	800
Dried wheat grass or barley grass	514
Sardines	443
Nori	260
Almonds	233
Parsley	203
Turnip greens	191
Sunflower seeds	174
Watercress	151
Garbonzo beans	150
Pinto beans	135
Kale	134
Spirulina	131
Collard greens	117
Sesame seeds	110
Chinese cabbage	106
Tofu	100
Walnuts	99
Okra	88
Brown rice	33
Halibut	13

CALCIUM INHIBITORS

1. Coffee, soft drinks, and diuretics
2. Excessive protein, especially meat (beef, pork, lamb)
3. Refined sugar or too much of any concentrated sweetener of sweet-flavored food
4. Alcohol, marijuana, cigarettes, and other intoxicants
5. Too little or too much exercise
6. Excess salt
7. The Solanum genus of vegetables-tomatoes in particular, but also potatoes, eggplant, and bell peppers contain calcium inhibitor solanine

Once the walls become thick and hard from years of buildup, nutrients cannot pass through freely. Vitamins will not make a difference in your health if they are not passing through the walls of your intestines. Moreover, all dairy products (even low fat milk) contain animal fat, which promotes heart disease.

Dark-green leafy foods have a 2-to-1 ratio of calcium to magnesium—the perfect ratio for absorbing minerals and keeping muscles working properly. For thousands of years, people have eaten greens because human stomachs, intestines, and livers recognize, digest, and assimilate this form of calcium and a variety of other wonderful minerals. I suggest romaine lettuce, turnip greens, alfalfa sprouts, dandelions, Swiss chard, beet tops, kale, clover sprouts, collard greens, and any of the wide variety of seaweeds such as kelp, or dulse, which all have an abundant supply of calcium, plus a variety of other helpful minerals. I always remind my patients that unless they are color-blind, it's easy to recognize a calcium food. That food will be green. Be careful though—this kind of a diet may just cause you to grow longer ears and a fluffy white tail!

The Sources of Calcium Chart lists sources of calcium, beginning with a few foods, such as sea vegetables, with which you may not be familiar. The Calcium Inhibitors Chart lists some of the foods that inhibit the body's absorption of calcium.

Green leafy vegetables, when eaten raw, have a very large cell wall that can't be easily broken down by the human enzymes that help us digest our food. We refer to this large cell as *roughage*—it is the "broom" in our colons that sweeps everything through and helps us maintain regular bowel movements. If we want to absorb more nutrients, we must break through the plant's cell wall with heat, but we must never let our vegetables touch boiling water unless we are making soups or stews. Vitamins found in dark, leafy greens are water-soluble. Once immersed in boiling water, vitamins are absorbed into the water and destroyed. The cooking method I recommend most often to my patients is steaming. A stainless steel or bamboo basket (both can be found in most grocery stores) will hold the greens above the boiling water and preserve the precious vitamins.

Herbal supplements are my second choice for calcium. After having looked over the food list, a calcium-mineral supplement might look more appealing. The hectic schedules of most working adults lend themselves to dark green herbs, whether wild or domestic, that have been dried and put in capsule form. These capsules contain a mixture of dandelions, alfalfa, red clover, blue-green algae, marshmallow roots, nettles, oat straw, plantain, and dulse and kelp (two kinds of seaweed rich in the minerals no longer found in our depleted farm soil). They are Mother Nature's pharmacy. I describe them as calcium minerals because they combine broad-spectrum minerals high in calcium with an evenly balanced supply of magnesium. The minerals found in these whole-food herbal supplements are perfectly balanced because they have been packaged as only Mother Nature can.

Manufactured supplements, such as calcium citrate, are my third choice for adding more calcium to the diet. Available at most quality health food stores, this supplement has a much better absorption rate than the calcium derived from oyster shells.

If you drink coffee each morning, do NOT take your calcium supplement at that time. Chocolate, black tea, caffeinated teas, cocoa, many soft drinks, diet pills, aspirin, various analgesics used for migraine headaches and vascular pain, and even some herbal preparations contain either caffeine or very closely related substances. (Examples of such elements are theogromine in chocolate and cocoa and theophylline in black tea.[7]) Caffeine interferes with the body's ability to absorb calcium, so taking it while ingesting caffeine is the same as throwing it away. For this reason, *I suggest taking mineral supplements in the evening.* Our bodies absorb minerals better while we sleep.

Our bodies are wonderful self-regulating mechanisms. When our backs are stiff or our shoulders continually tight, it is just their way of telling us that we are low on minerals—that there are not enough available calcium, magnesium, and micro-minerals to make our muscles work properly. This nutritional lack can cause heavy muscular spasms that pull spinal vertebrae (these bones that make up the spine) out of alignment, putting pressure, torque, or pinch on nerves that have to maneuver out through small openings in the vertebrae on their way to various organs. Low-back problems, headaches, muscle spasms in the legs, calcium spurring in the vertebrae, heel spurs—all can be attributed to calcium-mineral deficiencies. Menstrual pain can also be attributed to calcium-mineral deficiency. The uterine muscles contract continuously for three to five days of the menstrual cycle, so there is a much greater demand for minerals just before and during this time. At the first onset of menstrual pain and cramping, women need to increase—maybe even double—their normal calcium-mineral intake. And remember, the heart is a huge muscle, pumping again and again: its calcium-mineral requirements are very high.

All patients who walk into my office are evaluated to ascertain if their calcium-mineral levels are keeping up with their muscles' demands. For example, weight lifters need protein to build muscle mass, but without calcium, they will not be able to use those muscles once they are built. The same holds true for everyone. Whether you are a mother with small children or you sit in front of a computer all day, your muscles are working and need nutrition in the form of minerals to perform well. Doing the laundry, picking up the children, pushing doors open, or slamming drawers closed—it's all a simple matter of supply and demand. Are you supplying the nutrition to keep up the demands you make on your muscles?

I usually start every examination with a diet history that asks my patients if they support their activities and/or their lifestyles with plenty of dark-green leafy foods. If not, do they supplement with calcium? Half of my job is getting blood to the problem; the other half is a responsibility the patient must share, and that is knowing what's in their blood. If our chiropractors, massage therapists or even our medical doctors are not concerned with what we put in our mouths, they are not addressing our whole (*istic*) health problem. A good multiple vitamin is a great start. Look to your local health food store for the best quality vitamins and mineral supplements, but don't forget the greens!

---

1. *Eat Right, Live Longer* by Dr. Neil Bernard, M.D. Harmony Books, NY 1995 p. 168.

2. Zemel, M.B.: Phosphates and Calcium. *Journal of American Dietetic Association.* 81, (5): p. 606, 1982.

3. Massey, L.K., and Strong, M.M.: Soft Drink Consumption. Phosphorous Intake, and Osteoporosis, *Journal of American Dietetic Association.* 80, (6): p. 581, 1982.

4. Mash, A.G., Sanchez, T.V., Mickelson, O., Keiser, J., and Mayor, G.: Cortical Bone Density of Adult Lacto-ovo-vegetarians and Omnivorous Women. *Journal of American Dietetic Association.* 76: pp. 148-51, 1998; Calvo, M.S., Dietary Phosphorus, Calcium Metabolism, and Bone. *Journal of Nutrition.* 123: pp. 1627-33.

5. *Eat Right, Live Longer* by Dr. Neil Bernard, M.D. Harmony Books, NY 1995 p. 168.

6. *Nutrition and Diet Therapy*, By Sue Rodewell-Williams, 5th Edition, Times Mirror/Mosby College Publishing 1985 p. 170.

7. John Pitchford, *Healing with Whole Foods* (North Atlantic Books, 1993), 167.

Chapter 2

Muscle, Bone, and Naprapathy

A naprapath specializes in health problems that originate in the muscles, ligaments, and tendons—commonly referred to as the *soft connecting tissues.* A chiropractor specializes in *moving bone*— an approach originally based on the theory that all disease can be traced to the misalignment of the spinal column, which causes bones to be displaced. Bones are held in place by soft tissue. Any imbalance due to poor nutrition, worrying, trauma, or negative thinking causes these soft tissues to pull our bones out of position, and can result in the entire muscular-skeletal system losing its natural perfect alignment. Providing good nutrition to soft tissues so that they do not spasm, lock up, and pull our bones out of place is the first step before any bone adjustment is attempted.

The naprapath pays close attention to the state of the soft tissue, and uses slow and gentle massage-like techniques to pump blood into these areas. Naprapathic manipulation is done gently and easily so that the soft tissue lets the bone yield. If a bone adjustment is done quickly and dynamically, without proper preparation to the muscles, tendons, and ligaments, they may end up being strained.

If someone told you to touch your toes with your fingertips, would you dive down as hard and fast as you could to grab those toes? Or would you perhaps breathe deeply, do a few stretches and let the blood circulate around your muscles so that they can stretch and let you *ease* down? Naprapaths do not use dynamic thrusts, but apply gentle manipulation to ease the bone through its full range of possible motion. Thus, a basic difference between a naprapath and a chiropractor is one of velocity.

Tight shoulders are tight muscles that can pull the vertebrae out of alignment. A good naprapath will test the "bumpy" part of each vertebra, beginning at the back of the neck and descending between the wing bones—or scapula—all the way to the hips. This "bumpy" aspect of the spinal vertebrae is called the *spinus process*. [**Figures 2.1 and 2.2**] The spinus process can be painful on either the left or right side, and sometimes both. By placing the thumb and the first finger on opposite sides of each bone and pushing toward the middle, it can be determined if the vertebra is sore or tender. A fall as a child, wrestling with one's older brother, or any spinal injury can make one vertebra sore to the touch, and the very next one not painful at all.

The naprapathic theory is that the painful side is the buckled tissue side. The other side, which is tighter and usually painless, is over-tightened connecting tissue that needs to be stretched. The angle to stretch changes with the position of each vertebrae. [**Figure 2.3**]

Because of the way each vertebra is stacked on top of the next, a naprapathic professional needs to analyze pain levels and apply a slow, massage-like stretch whenever a tender vertebra is found. Usually, the side that elicits pain also has deep soreness in those muscles on the same side of the spine. The naprapath applies long stretching massage techniques to the muscles, lateral pulling motions, and even little circular massage-type strokes in order to pump

Figure 2.1 - Spinal vertebrae intervertebral disc

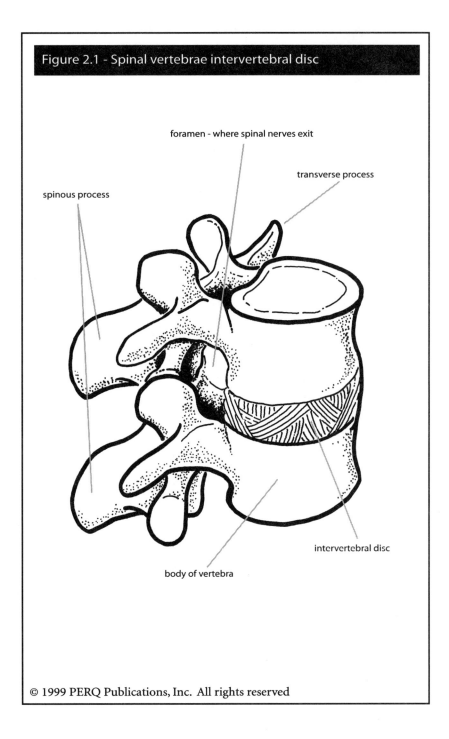

foramen - where spinal nerves exit

transverse process

spinous process

intervertebral disc

body of vertebra

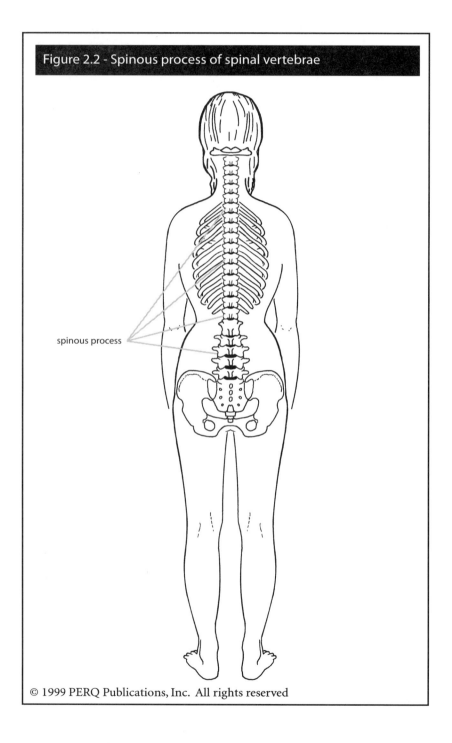

Figure 2.2 - Spinous process of spinal vertebrae

spinous process

blood into the sore tissue. This is an important first step prior to bone manipulation. In addition to buckled fibers, soreness also can be linked to a lack of oxygen and nutrient-filled blood at the affected area. By massaging all the muscles, tendons, and ligaments that surround the bones, I pump as much blood in there as possible. The entire treatment usually begins with 10 to 15 minutes of hot packs to promote circulation. A cessation of pain means that blood has circulated throughout the area, the desirable result. Less torque on the bone and more blood to the surrounding tissues means more comfort for the patient.

Rub a Little Longer

Although the treatment feels like a great massage, it is not painless. When tension is high, circulation between the fibers of the soft tissue is poor, and they accumulate toxins. When the naprapath pushes, moves, or jiggles this tissue in order to increase circulation, fresh blood floods in and the toxins are washed out into the circulatory system. The release of these poisons can cause a "healing crisis"—headaches and muscle soreness later that evening or even the next day. But no pain, no gain! The health benefits after that initial treatment far outweigh that first little soreness.

How George Got Sore

I was in the second year of my naprapathic studies, with a manipulation class or two under my belt, when I successfully convinced my Uncle George, who'd been complaining about a bad back, to agree to a sample treatment. I put Uncle George face down on the den floor and gave him a treatment without first warning him that the treatment might make him sore. Old, stagnated, devitalized blood can be locked inside in the areas of tightly-held tension. That blood is pure poison, and once it is moved into normal circulation, those poisons can make you hurt. I was unaware that I must warn patients—not once, but twice—that they might suffer some painful detoxifying aftereffects from naprapathic manipulation.

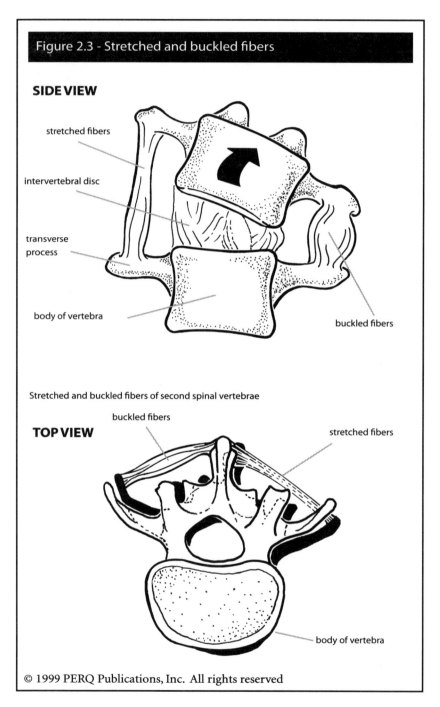

Figure 2.3 - Stretched and buckled fibers

SIDE VIEW

stretched fibers

intervertebral disc

transverse process

body of vertebra

buckled fibers

Stretched and buckled fibers of second spinal vertebrae

TOP VIEW

buckled fibers

stretched fibers

body of vertebra

That's exactly what happened to Uncle George. I only heard years later that he was tremendously sore from that first treatment—so much so that, from that day to this, he has never asked for another. But if he had returned a second time, he wouldn't have experienced that same pain. By then, most of the poisons would have been cleared away. Thank you, Uncle George. From then on, I never forgot to tell my patients that it's normal to be sore after the initial treatment.

Although all those poisons need to clear away for health to resume, you can keep the effects to a minimum by following these recommendations:

1   **Drink eight glasses of water at room temperature throughout the entire day after the first treatment.** This dilutes the toxins and helps the circulating blood flush stagnated accumulations away. Mixing a little apple cider vinegar (approximately one half to one teaspoon) in a glass of water two or three times a day after the treatment also helps.

2   **Soak in a warm bath with either one or two cups of Epsom salts (high in magnesium), or one or two cups of Masada bath salts (calcium-rich minerals scraped from the bottom of the Dead Sea and available from your local health food store).** For centuries, people have sought out hot mineral springs to bathe in their soothing waters. The heat opens up the pores and allows calcium, magnesium and trace minerals to enter and provide calming nutrients to the muscles and joints. In addition, the heat promotes circulation of fresh blood throughout the body's sore areas.

Here again, you can add one to two cups of apple cider vinegar to the bath water—apple cider vinegar and ONLY apple cider vinegar is very alkalinizing.

You might end up smelling like a salad, but once the
vinegar is in the body, it will greatly reduce the soreness or stiffness resulting from a treatment. A Masada
bath (my favorite scent is lavender, which promotes
joy in aromatherapy) once a week or following the
initial treatment is my standard recommendation.
In addition, both Epsom and Masada salts are excellent for relieving soreness after a weekend spent
stretching and straining muscles that haven't had the
proper nutrition to do that extra work.

3. **Use Zheng Gu Shui, a Chinese liniment spray to
   prevent soreness.** I automatically give all my new
   patients a bottle of this liniment, but Icy Hot and
   Ben-Gay™ are also effective. These products stimulate new blood to flush the troubled area and push
   the toxic accumulations out.

So, Uncle George, I apologize for making you sore and I'm sorry
that you had to be the sacrificial lamb—but think of all the people
you've helped!

Getting the Blood There—Hot Packs or Cold Packs?

One of the questions I'm most frequently asked is when to use heat
and when to use ice. At the first sign of injury, the body, in its infinite wisdom, tries to isolate the problem area by creating a welt, or
weal, that surrounds the injured site and walls off the injury and
inflammation. Because there is heating, swelling, and pain going
on inside this big red bump, a standard medical recommendation
is to first apply an ice pack, which allows the body to limit the amount
of swelling. Keeping that ball of inflammation as small as possible
with a little ice will mean a much smaller clean-up job later as the
body attempts to heal the area. But after about 15 minutes, the body's
protective mechanism says, "Wait a minute. This is way too cold
for our tissues. I'd better warm that area up or I'm going to have
some frostbite down there!" The body reacts to the excessive cold
by attempting to return warmth to the injured area, creating the

opposite effect of what was intended. After 15 minutes, the cold pack should be removed for 30 to 45 minutes, and then applied again for another 15 minutes. This on-and-off procedure can be repeated for up to 24 hours after sustaining an injury.

After the first 24 hours, the injured area needs to be heated. A hot pack brings in blood containing cells that eat up the products causing inflammation. This blood also contains healing elements, minerals and oxygen. After 20 to 30 minutes, the injured area needs to be cooled off. This moves the debris-filled blood away from the injury. Alternating heat and cold is the oldest therapy known.

Heat can be applied with a hot pack, a moist heating pad, a hot water bottle wrapped in towels, or by massage or naprapathic-chiropractic manipulation. The after-cooling can be accomplished with ice or a rubefacient ("rube" means *red*—the redness from the congested blood—"facient" refers to the skin), such as the Zheng Gu Shui liniment I use in my practice. Icy Hot, Ben-Gay, and Tiger Balm are also considered effective rubefacients. However, the simplest method is to remove the hot pack. This makes the skin cooler than the inner core of the body and allows the blood to redistribute itself back into the circulatory system, and that's our goal. Heating brings blood; cooling takes away surplus debris and excess swelling. As the swelling leaves, new blood rich in healing elements fills in behind it. Any product classified as a rubefacient produces this kind of circular action.

All too often, patients use their heating pads for hours or all night long. While this approach temporarily lessens or removes the pain, the pain is worse when they take the pad off. Hours of heat causes so much blood to accumulate that the entire injured area becomes engorged and drainage is poor. Moreover, the nerve endings are so compressed with extra fluid that they fire off pain signals left and right. The excess blood and fluid must be removed, and that can only occur if the area is cooled. Applying a rubefacient causes the congested blood to come up the surface of the skin because the skin is now cooler than the body.

This congested blood will migrate back into the body by a different path while new healing blood rushes into the injured area.

If you apply another round of hot packs after cool-down, wash off any rubefacients applied earlier. They are not meant to be covered tightly and heated a second time. When using Zheng Gu Shui just before bed to keep the circulation flowing while you sleep, there is normally no need to wash it off. One of my patients related a very amusing story. She applied Zheng Gu Shui to her lower back just before going to bed. She used a little too much and it flowed down between her buttocks. When her husband became a little amorous later, the Zheng Gu Shui got into areas that were most uncomfortable for them both. Though not dangerous, their passion and the liniment resulted in quite a hot, memorable encounter.

Hot and Cold Water

Hot and cold therapy can sometimes be done with water. When an area is tight, stiff, or needs additional circulation, stand in a hot shower. Adjust the water as hot as you can stand it, and let it run on your neck and shoulders for three to four minutes. Then switch to cool or cold water for thirty seconds. Flushing the muscles with blood and then draining the blood in this manner should be repeated a couple of times in succession. If you stretch afterward, you will have better range of motion. I do *not*, however, recommend this therapy for anyone with serious heart disease and/or vascular insufficiency to the brain.

Some medical professionals recommend ending the hot/cold therapy on cold. But because some people tend to be very cold and others tend to be very warm, I suggest ending this shower technique on whichever temperature is more comfortable. If an injury seems to be getting worse after five minutes of applying heat, switch and apply cold instead. The objective is to lessen the pain and increase the range of motion. Listen to your body and experiment, whether in the shower or using hot and cold packs. Taking responsibility for your health means first listening to the advice of a qualified healer, then using your own inner voice to direct you to whatever sounds reasonable.

Now that I've told you the hot and cold of things, I'm going to change the rules. Some patients come in with an injury—a bump on the arm, a bruised finger, or a strained leg due to a fall. They are different from those patients who wake up with mysterious aches and pains, or whose backs go out when they bend down to pick up a piece of paper. With this latter group, the problem often stems from lack of sufficient mineral nutrients (especially calcium) for the workload they've taken on, whether they've started a new exercise program or they've been doing a lot of lifting. In this case, I heat the patient's site of inflammation immediately after the injury or as soon as the stiffness appears. Take a bath in Masada bath salts is my first recommendation. Applying hot packs to the painful area for 20 minutes also proves very helpful. This increases the circulation and raises the nutrient levels, which often eases the stiffness or muscle spasms and decreases the pain components.

Sometimes the workload hasn't increased but the person is emotionally distressed. Gary was a patient whose 15-year-old stepson tried to commit suicide. At the time, Gary was on a business trip and had to fly home. He sat on a plane for eight hours, agonizing over the boy's mental state. The more Gary worried, the more his muscles tensed. In addition, eating restaurant food had lowered Gary's available calcium-mineral levels. When he reached down to pick up a paper two weeks later, it was inevitable that his back "simply went out."

There is always a logical, easily understood reason why our backs, necks, or hips start out stiff in the morning and get worse as the day goes on. We need to examine our diets and ascertain how much meat and carbonated beverages we've consumed, robbing ourselves of calcium minerals. We need to recall how much muscle work we've done. No matter how much it turns out to be, heating any area delivers more blood, and with blood comes all the necessary nutrients.

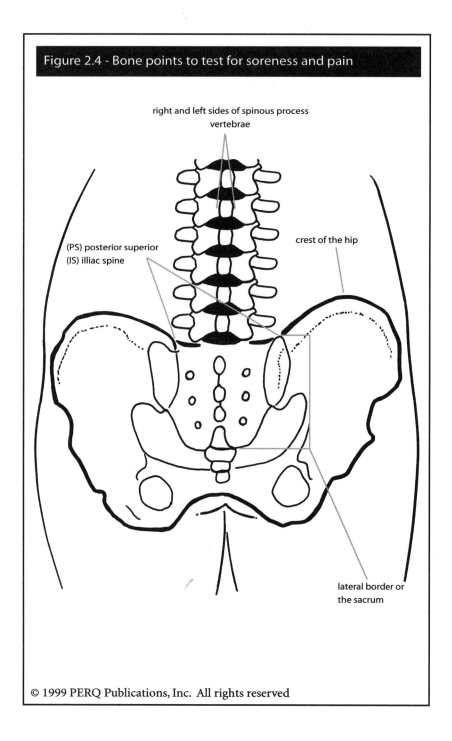

Figure 2.4 - Bone points to test for soreness and pain

Protective Muscle Spasms

Occasionally, we strain a muscle or joint, and the body knows that if we move again we'll strain those fibers even more. In response, the body will develop a protective muscle spasm, usually in the muscles along the spine. The spasm encourages the muscles in the troubled area to hold so tightly that we end up walking with a definite crook—bent over to one side or the other. By immobilizing us somewhat, muscle spasms save us from even more serious injury.

On these occasions, patients need to listen to their body very carefully. If their backs have immobilized them and they can't walk, then they should sit. If they can't sit, they should lie down. People who are continually on the go to avoid being with themselves should understand that inner spiritual truth is revealed when we sit quietly and listen to our inner voices. We should quiet our minds and listen to our bodies. I always tell my patients that their disease patterns are exactly what they seem. If they are experiencing trouble with their eyes, perhaps they are avoiding seeing the truth. Children with constant ear infections may be shutting out the surrounding chatter in their environments.

To be in touch with our bodies, we must pay attention. When our heels hurt, we must pay attention. When we have persistent gas, bloating, or digestive problems, we must pay attention. When an ear itches or when we suffer from athlete's foot, we must pay attention. Nothing happens in isolation within the body—everything is part of a disease *complex*. Look at the disease, be with it, be part of it, think about it, understand what it feels like. Spend some time with your disease pattern, and then ask yourself what it reminds you of. When did you feel this way as a child? What childhood story does the sitting, lying down, or inability to walk remind you of? Your pattern of disease-discomfort comes again and again till you get it right , so do not just think, "My back hurts," or "I have a bad back." Think the whole thing through. Only then should you decide to move on and give up those patterns.

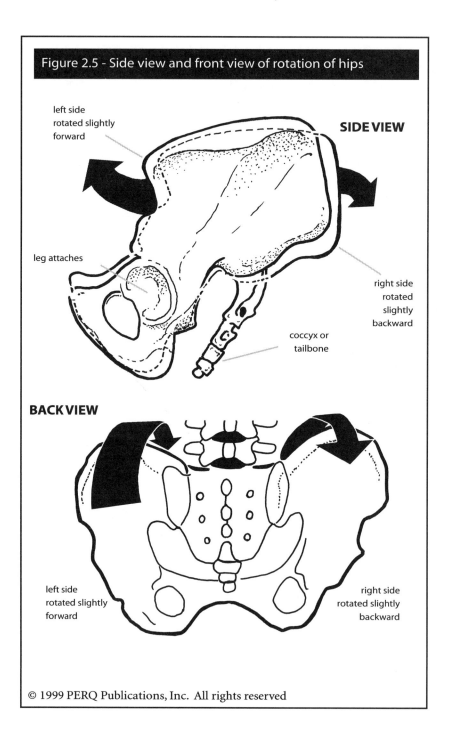

Figure 2.5 - Side view and front view of rotation of hips

left side rotated slightly forward

SIDE VIEW

leg attaches

right side rotated slightly backward

coccyx or tailbone

BACK VIEW

left side rotated slightly forward

right side rotated slightly backward

Testing Bony Vertebrae

Out of a hundred patients who walk into my office and are asked whether their low-back problem is on the right or left, a hundred say it's in the middle. But it's the naprapathic chiropractor's job to discover where the problem really exists. After palpation (touching) of each side of each vertebra in the pelvis and lower back, I always find that the problem is on one side or the other— *never* in the middle.

The support system for the vertebrae, or bony points, consists of connective tissue—tendon, ligaments, and muscle. [**Figure 2.4**] To analyze these points and their connective tissues, I apply the naprapathic theory of stretched and buckled fibers. The side of a vertebra that is painful to the touch is the side where the tissue is buckled or compressed. This is Mother Nature's alarm system, so we don't want any aspirin to deaden our pain response. On the opposite side of this vertebra, the connective tissue is usually very tight, so this side needs to be stretched. When pain is found on both sides, I must ascertain which side is the more painful—or which side becomes more painful as I continue to push on it. Then I know that the opposite side needs stretching.

You can perform this examination yourself by doing a little poking and prodding where the vertebrae meet the hips. The picture shows some of the areas to which you can apply a little pressure to analyze which side is more painful.

Oh No! One of Your Legs is Shorter than the Other— Guess What? Everyone's is!

Now that we have analyzed the position and level of pain of each spinal vertebra, let's look at the large bones that make up your hips. These bones do not normally appear symmetrical while standing straight. [**Figure 2.5**] I refer to this as the normal hip rotation. At the bottom of the lumbar spine, where the hips meet the back, you will find the L4 and L5 vertebrae and the first sacral vertebra, S1. Most disc problems occur between the fourth and/or fifth lumbar vertebrae and the first sacral. This is because an incredible amount of torque and tension surrounds the lower lumbar, the sacral, and the junction of the hip bones, also called *os innominata* or literally the nameless bone. The entire weight of the upper body rests on this pivotal point where the connecting tissues attach the spine firmly to the hip structure.

Crossing our legs can affect the hip rotation. Most people always cross the same leg over the knee of the other leg. Right-handed people tend to cross the right leg over the left knee. Left-handed folks can go either way. And although it's not a hard and fast rule, if we sleep on our sides, this leg-crossing pattern continues. Judge for yourself. Lie on either side in a casual sleeping position. Bring the right leg toward your chest, just an inch or two higher than the left leg, and hold that position for three to five minutes. Then switch, bringing the left leg higher than the right. The more comfortable position is probably how you are accustomed to sleeping, and that pattern is usually continued during the day when you cross your legs.

Why does crossing the legs influence the hip rotation? As the knee comes up, the same-side hip bone shifts back. The upper thigh bone also shifts back and a little lower which, in turn, shifts the lower leg bones down. The result of the altered hip position makes one leg appear shorter than the other. Because we all have natural hip rotation, every person who walks into my office has this discrepancy. If we continually cross the same leg over the same knee and continually sleep in that position for approximately five out of eight hours each night, we stretch all the connecting tissues on one side of the hips. Because the bones are held in a ring structure surrounding our pelvic organs, the other side of the hips will move forward. What affects one side influences the other.

You can judge the amount of discrepancy in leg length by placing a person face down with their head straight. Then wrap your palm around the front of the ankle so that your middle finger rests on the bone that pokes out on the inside of the ankle. You can see approximately what kind of leg-length difference exists. A normal

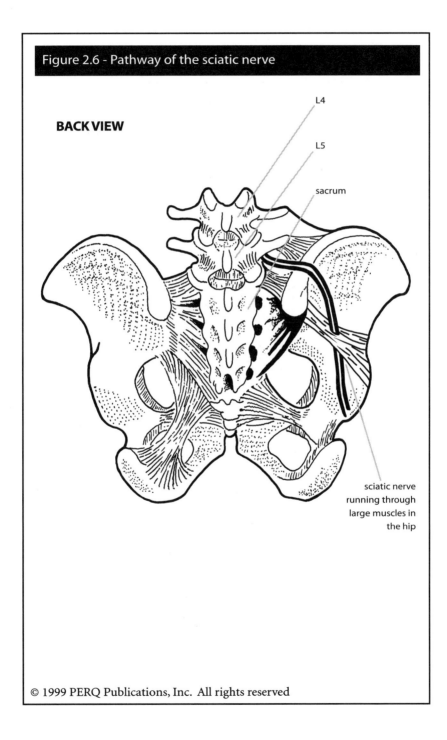

Figure 2.6 - Pathway of the sciatic nerve

BACK VIEW

L4

L5

sacrum

sciatic nerve running through large muscles in the hip

discrepancy is one-quarter inch or less. But if the hips are in a tight spasm that pulls one hip higher in order to protect the lower spinal nerves from being painfully sparked, you can often see a greater difference in leg lengths. If there is more than one-quarter inch difference when the ankles are placed side by side, then a problem exists in the hips that needs naprapathic-chiropractic treatment.

With rotated hips and leg-length discrepancies greater than a quarter of an inch, the first priority is to relax any existing muscle spasm. (Occasionally, a muscle spasm is present as a means of protecting an already inflamed nerve so that we don't turn or twist the wrong way and irritate it further.) Calcium minerals will relax the muscle spasm, and may also stop the nerve irritation—as always, healing starts with good nutrition. Although this is not what your MD wants to prescribe, it will effectively heal the problem when the doctor's prescription for muscle relaxers has run out and the spasm returns. Drugs (what natural healers call "Band-Aid therapy") that stop the symptoms but don't address the cause always lead back to natural medicine. Meanwhile, an orthopedic support belt from your local pharmacy can stabilize the back, preventing movement in a manner that would further irritate sensitive tissue.

Muscle and Nerve Irritation—Sciatica

When physicians analyze pain and spasms in the nerves and muscles of our lower backs, it is impossible for them to separate muscle from nerve. As the nerves exit the vertebrae, they pass through ligament and muscle tissue. The large nerve that exits the bottom of the spine is called the sciatic nerve. As it runs through the large muscles of the buttocks (*i.e.*, the *gluteus maximus, gluteus medius, gluteus minimus,* and the *piriformis*), any muscle tension or spasm can irritate the sciatic nerve, causing it to spark pain signals at the point of the problem in the lower back or anywhere along its path. This can include the thigh, knee, calf, or any part of the foot. [**Figures 2.6 and 2.7**] Radiating pain caused by a nerve from the lower back is commonly called sciatica, and it often does what-

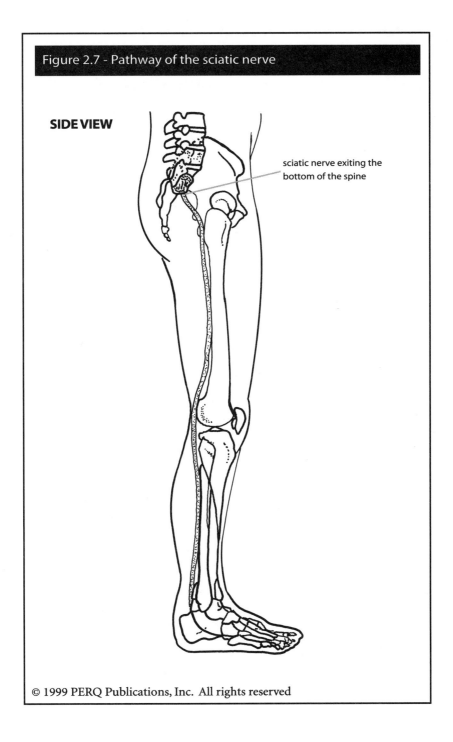

Figure 2.7 - Pathway of the sciatic nerve

SIDE VIEW

sciatic nerve exiting the bottom of the spine

ever it wants to do. Its pain pattern can skip the thigh and be felt only in the lower leg, or can appear in any combination of the above-mentioned locations. One day you can experience calf pain, and the next your toes are numb and your lower back hurts so much you're afraid to move.

When sciatica occurs, it's important for the healer to analyze which muscles, joints, and bones are involved. Patients will be asked in what position they are most comfortable; if they experience pain when standing, sitting, and/or lying down; whether the pain is less as they stand or sit; where the pain is located; and what action sets it off.

When sciatic nerve irritation accompanies a low-back problem, pain impulses can either travel up or down the nerve, or stay in one particular spot and bypass another area. I repeatedly see patients who experience pain on the side of their calf even though the restriction, or point of the original problem, occurs up in the lower back. The pattern of nerve irritation lets me know which nerve is involved. If the pain is coming around the front of the groin, we are dealing with the L3 nerve coming out of the third lumbar vertebra. If the pain pattern comes around the front of the thigh down to the knee, again L3. If the nerve pain comes around to the lateral, or on the outside of the calf, then the L4, or fourth lumbar vertebra, is involved. And if it hits the top of the foot, the fifth lumbar vertebra is suspect.

Massaging the muscles of the lower back parallel to the suspect vertebrae (once a day for five minutes) at home is an excellent means of promoting good circulation and may be very helpful with low-back pain. However, any more than once a day may exacerbate the problem. A naprapathic-chiropractic treatment is usually given one to three times a week. Deep massage breaks apart congestion held in tight stiff painful areas. If the massage is too heavy, it can break the channels in the lymphatic system that remove debris from a site of inflammation. Occasionally, the inability to move this debris causes the soreness patients feel after their initial treatment.

The new blood that rushes in to the massaged area removes excess fluids, dead cells, and other debris from the inflammation. Thus, it is important to give the body time to remove all the debris that's been churned up by the massage—usually a day to a day and a half. A hot bath followed by a cooling liniment will help this along. The hot bath helps move fresh blood in; the liniment helps move debris-filled blood out (we're back to hot and cold therapy again). This simply gives the body, a wonderful natural healer in itself, the chance to do its job. At home, a little peanut oil is great for this muscle massage. Between treatments, let hot and cold water therapy help remove the debris you've churned up.

I always recommend soft-tissue muscle massage surrounding the area of pain (e.g., the whole hip, the lower back, and the thigh of the affected side), and also massage the hip, lower back, and thigh of the unaffected side. A naprapathic-chiropractic treatment needs to leave the body balanced. Both sides need their energy flow. If one side of the body is sore, has an irritated nerve or is experiencing muscle spasms, the other side reacts by holding tight and doing extra muscle work. It is amazing how much extra muscle work the body performs merely trying to avoid re-injury. Thus, I never work just one side of the body.

I also recommend B-complex if the nerve is irritated down any part of the leg. Specifically, I use Complete B-Complex by Rainbow Light. You may have to ask the health food store manager to order it, but it's worth the extra trouble. (Chapter 6 explores in more depth nerve problems, foods that irritate nerves, and foods that strengthen them.)

Chapter 3

Lower Back and "Lower"

My Low-Back Injury

During the twelve years I've treated low-back pain, I've been very lucky to have only strained my own back on one occasion. Unlike most people, my emotional response to each new injury is almost one of excitement. I'm not asking the Great Spirit for any more illnesses than I'm obliged to get, but it is a wonderful way for me to step inside the bodies of my patients, to really feel where their pain begins, and how their pain patterns change as they recover. Being injured allows me to see how points of massage and manipulation affect the whole hip and low-back structures and also to try the remedies I recommend to my patients.

I am a polo player and love the sport to the point of obsession. I was riding in my very first women's outdoor tournament on a grass field when I injured my lower back. The field, which is 900 yards long by 300 yards wide, is three times the size of an indoor field. And because the speeds are tremendous, there must be complete trust between rider and horse. The animal is 70 percent of the game: if it can't get you there, you can't make the shot. So, if you have any fear of going fast or are worried about stopping the animal you're riding, those fears are doubled and tripled on an outdoor grass field. To say I was nervous is an understatement.

My horse was saddled and his legs wrapped for protection from swinging mallets. With helmet, knee pads, and my best polo mallet, I was ready to take my horse, Allegro, to circle the field and hit a couple of practice balls. Polo players ride with four reins (two on each side of the horse's mouth) that are interlaced between the four fingers of the left hand. I, however, could not manage to get those four reins between my fingers. I had done it a hundred times, but I was so tense that even this fundamental exercise was beyond my control.

Finally, I got it right. I took the first shot, and "Yow!" I strained the muscles that keep my buttocks in the saddle (technically, the muscles that attach the upper leg, or femur, to the hips—the ilium bones). I was devastated. Quickly, I pointed Allegro toward my car on the sidelines. After my teammates helped me off the horse, I rummaged through my trunk, which normally holds every remedy I own. I found treatments for coughs and colds, pills for diabetics, a Chinese mixture for female problems, and finally a bottle of Chinese liniment for muscle strains with half a squirt left in it. I poured it on my spastic hip, wishing to the Great Spirit that I had some peanut oil to rub into the muscle. I was hoisted back up onto Allegro and, amazingly enough, was able to play the entire tournament without pain.

I played like lightning, with amazing back-handed shots, incredibly accurate shots-on-the-goal, and even an under-the-horse's-neck shot while leaning half out of the saddle. My team won, but could I get down off Allegro? No! I had done exactly what I tell every one of my weekend-warrior patients not to do—continue to play once they've been hurt. Listen to the body: it is wise and will tell you when to stop. My body protected me from feeling pain, but I could barely move my hip. I had to be hoisted off Allegro and into my car, and, as the stiffness got worse, I was forced to drive home using my left foot.

Once home, I applied Zheng Gu Shui liniment, massaged with both olive and peanut oils, took hot Masada baths, and ingested double and triple doses of calcium-minerals. I babied myself for three days before I got that hip back to aching and limping. Normal was another week away.

I will always remember that low-back sprain. I will never forget exactly which tissues can consistently bind up and entrap the sciatic nerve, and I know precisely where to rub and how to gently rotate the large hip bones. If a patient walks into my office with sciatica, I know exactly the path that nerve travels, how it becomes irritated, and what the pain feels like. I've been there. I am one with my patients.

Get in the Car the Right Way, Please!
Do you experience pain when getting in or out of a car? Most people put one foot in the car first, sit down on the seat, and then bring in the other foot. This approach is not good for the lower back because it has a tendency to "go out" when the upper body and lower body are moving in two different directions at the same time. Other activities that put the body in the position to strain the lower back—especially if there has been a previous history of low-back pain—include golfing, waxing the car, vacuuming, sweeping, raking, and shoveling snow. Even when we pick up a piece of paper, we twist at the waist, again causing our bodies to move in two different directions at once. So, the next time you enter a car, first stand with your back to the side of the seat, sit down, then swing both legs into the car together.

Chronic Low-Back Pain
The Heat of a Low-Back Strain - Cooling Foods and Herbs
Many people come to see me simply because they've strained their lower backs. Their muscle fibers spasm (causing a tight stiff

feeling), creating tension on the nerves that exit the spinal column. However, it is often impossible to differentiate between the nerve and the muscle as the source of the problem unless we cut the patient open and dissect the tissue. A little too severe, you say? Both problems are solved with essential nutrition: calcium-mineral for the muscle and B-complex for the nerve. With a few treatments, most people are fine.

Other patients come in with pain patterns that resemble a simple strain; however, they have moved past that point and actually are in the chronic phase, where the strain has become continuous. The bone has been torqued for such a long time that now joint and bone interplay, and the position of the disc, are all showing signs of wear.

Technically, *chronic* means that a medical problem has existed for more than three weeks. Most patients do very well with manipulation, but occasionally, manipulation can make some chronic low-back problems worse. Of course, I'm not referring to the initial treatment, which can leave them a little sore. But if the pain pattern increases without relief after four treatments, Chinese theory suggests that the problem area is so hot that it needs to be cooled. An inflammation at the site of an injury normally feels hot to the touch, and the "heat" that patients eat makes the heat in their backs worse. In this instance, "heat" is defined as food that is either hot and spicy, dry, crispy, burnt, or of animal origin.

A live animal has an inherent temperature that is transferred to anyone eating that animal's flesh. This concept of heat is also associated with any food that is generally lacking in moisture. A good example is toast, which carries more heat than bread. Even the crust of a slice of untoasted bread carries more heat than the center of the slice. I always say that little kids who cut the crust off their bread are instinctively managing the internal heating mechanisms of their bodies. In other words, the wisdom of our unconscious acts perpetuates the body's natural mechanisms to maintain health.

When chronic low-back pain exists, take a good look at the patient's diet to see if there is an excess of heating foods present. I say excess because every diet needs a balance of warming and cooling foods, but when the fire in your low back rages for too long, eliminate some of the foods that might cause increased heating. Try cooling fruits and raw and steamed vegetables. However, some tropical fruits, which are grown in hot climates, convey heat and should be avoided [**See Warm and Cold Properties Foods Charts, on page 38, for those fruits**]. In addition, adults can take cooling herbs, such as echinacea or astragalus in doses of four to six capsules, two hundred-fifty to five hundred milligrams each, per day for one week.

While you are attempting to cool the fire with diet, I recommend hot and cold alternating water therapies or Masada baths, followed by the liniment Zheng Gu Shui. Special attention is needed to avoid hot, spicy foods. **Pepper** makes joint pain hot and fiery.

Aimee was an excellent example of too much heat. She was studying intensely in her last year of law school. Taking extra time to cook well-rounded meals would have taken away from study time so, often chips and hot salsa became a quick meal. Eventually salsa was added to eggs, meats, and vegetables. The heart needs a fiery intensity to work long hours for extended periods of time. Unconsciously, she was using the false heat from the salsa to create a great fire to drive her heart for the long hours of study, but that heat was making the joints in her feet and hips hot. I gave her the herb ginseng that delivers energy and intensity to the heart and took her off all the salsa. Withdrawal was not easy but within a couple of weeks the joint pain disappeared. A warm- and cold-propertied foods chart given to me by Dr. Lau, my traditional Chinese physician, is shown on page 38.

It takes a trained professional to determine whether this excessive heat situation actually exists. The naprapathic-chiropractor uses diet, physical symptoms, and occasionally X-rays to analyze the patient's condition. X-rays help us look inside the body to evaluate the level of deterioration of bone and to judge the spacing

WARM PROPERTIES FOODS

warm drinks	vegetables		meats	grain
warm water	peapod	scallion	sausage	bread
tea	cabbage	potatoes	shrimp	noodle
coffee	cauliflower	green bean	chicken	egg
	spinach	pumpkin	crab	rice
	broccoli	celery	pork	
fruit	water chestnut	onion	beef	**other**
grape	bamboo shoot	eggplant	squid	honey
apple		asparagus	lobster	
strawberry orange	peanut	green onion	duck	
dates	soybean corn	sweet potato	oyster	
papaya	parsley	taro	fish	
	pea	napa	ham	
			turkey	

COLD PROPERTIES FOODS

cold drinks	fruit	vegetables		beans
ice water	cantaloupe	bok-choy	mushroom	to-fu
coke	honey dew	turnip	lettuce	mung beans
apple juice	banana	cucumber		kidney beans
orange juice	bitter melon	sprout		lima beans
carrot juice	tomato	radish		soybeans
cranberry juice	grapefruit	watercress		
7-up	water-melon	seaweed		**dairy**
beer, etc.		eggplant		ice-cream
		barley		milk
		carrot		

between the bones where the disc lies. But, X-rays take a picture of only the hard tissues, while the disc that lies between each spinal vertebra is made up of soft tissue. Thus, the size of the disc is actually determined by the *spacing* between each bone. Further evaluation as to the health of the disc is done with magnetic resonance imaging (MRI).

The Chiropractic "Pop"

Naprapathic treatments, which are gentle and massage-like, do not generally irritate the back. Even these gentle pressures do not mean that the patient's back is silent. Supply an individual with plenty of minerals, approximately six glasses of good quality water, and regular stretching exercises, and any back can make noise when adjusted. Actually, that "pop" or audible "snap" has more to do with air than with bone. Each joint has a specific and limited range of motion. It can only open so wide. On either side of that possible opening is elastic tissue, called the elastic barrier of the joint. The manipulation stretches the joint open a little bit more, stressing the elastic. When the elastic reaches its maximum stretched point, air (actually a gas) rushes into the space, resulting in a popping sound. It is not a bone being moved into place, but actually air moving into a space that was previously occupied by elastic tissue.

Your Feet Never Lie

Because every point on the bottom of the foot relates to a point on the rest of the body (all low-back problems are reflected in the heels), [**Figure 3.1**] I begin every treatment with a thorough massage of the patient's feet. Sore or tender points give me a clue where to look for deficiencies and indicate which muscles or organs may be showing early signs of disease. By the same token, if the heel points that refer to the lower back are not sensitive or painful, I know that the low-back problem is not that serious. It probably only involves the muscles or maybe tendons and has not yet affected any joints or discs.

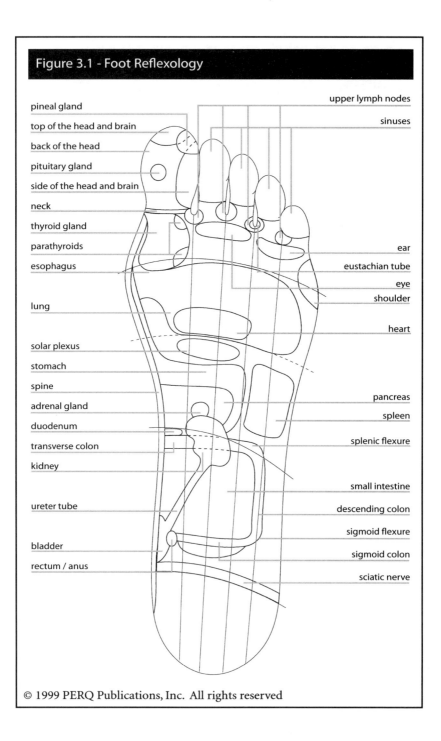

Figure 3.1 - Foot Reflexology

pineal gland

top of the head and brain

back of the head

pituitary gland

side of the head and brain

neck

thyroid gland

parathyroids

esophagus

lung

solar plexus

stomach

spine

adrenal gland

duodenum

transverse colon

kidney

ureter tube

bladder

rectum / anus

upper lymph nodes

sinuses

ear

eustachian tube

eye

shoulder

heart

pancreas

spleen

splenic flexure

small intestine

descending colon

sigmoid flexure

sigmoid colon

sciatic nerve

I examine the medial or inner side of the heels. If the right hip is sore, I usually find some soreness in the right heel (pain patterns usually occur on the same side of the body). If you spend the whole day on your feet, and one heel is much more sore than the other, it is a good indication that (1) you need to get off your feet, (2) you need to add minerals to support the muscle work that the lower back has been doing, and/or (3) the hip rotation has been stressed and could use a good treatment to realign the hips.

What does it mean to realign? Earlier I referred to normal hip rotation, which allows one hip to move forward while the other moves back. This rotation affects the back and the length of the leg. However, soft-tissue muscle spasms displace this normal movement. A good naprapathic-chiropractic treatment pumps blood into these tissues by massaging around the hip bones, the sacrum, and the individual bones of the spine that connect the hips to the lower back and then up the back, relieving some of these spasms. Manipulation becomes much more effective then, and the hips will go back to their normal rotation naturally. The hips, knees, ankles, and feet will be in alignment. This should decrease the uneven pressure on the heels and alleviate the pain.

Our knees often become problematic when the hips are rotated further than our normal quarter inch or so. When low-back discomfort increases, we torque our hips in an unnatural manner and begin to walk with an awkward gait in an effort to avoid more pain. Not only do the knees hurt, they can begin to making popping noises. Many patients have said, "You know, Doc, this knee not only hurts, but every time I take a step, it pops." Popping knees mean that the body's pH, or acid-base balance, has fallen more to the acidic side. Too much acidic food (*e.g.,* meats, fish, poultry, eggs, most dairy, refined sugars), as well as the acid found in drugs and chemicals, makes us prone to disease and infections. We need to add more base-side or alkalinizing foods, including fruits, vegetables, and sprouts to our diets. I also recommend adding apple cider vinegar—one teaspoon in a glass of water, taken two to three times a day. Only apple cider vinegar will change the body's pH toward its optimal alkalinized state.

Damaging the Discs of the Lower Back

Todd was a fireman when he walked into my office, and is still a fireman today, but only because he trusted the healing power of his own body.

Todd came into my office a couple of hours after seeing an orthopedic surgeon who wanted to put him in the hospital that same day to perform surgery. Part of the disc between his last two lumbar vertebrae, L4 and L5, had popped backwards where it did not belong, causing tremendous pain—mostly down Todd's leg.

Discs are like plump little cushions, mostly composed of water, that lie between each vertebra. The disc has a ball of gelatinous substance (the nucleus pulposus) in the center, with concentric rings surrounding it, holding the ball in place. [**Figure 3.2**] It functions like a hydraulic shock absorber, pulling together the bones above and below with the rings, while maintaining the distance between bones with the pressure in the ball. Imagine a balloon that is not inflated completely lying between your palms. As your fingers come closer together, the balloon pops out toward the back. As your thumbs get closer together, the balloon pops out toward the back and side. The gelatinous ball inside the disc tends to move away from the direction you bend, while still maintaining that needed cushion between the bones.

There are approximately 18 annular rings surrounding the ball. When we strain our backs picking up heavy objects, or when we carry heavy objects away from the center of our bodies, the tension on the ball is tremendous and puts incredible tension on the concentric rings. With continual lifting, we can break some of the fibers of those rings and, in the beginning, never show any symptoms. However, as more rings break down, it is more likely that the ball and the whole disc will bulge back and bump into the very sensitive tissues that lie behind and to the side of the disc. [**Figure 3.3**] These tissues have nerve fibers running through them that can spark with a great deal of pain. When this condition exists, and we continue to lift heavy objects, it will only get worse. More

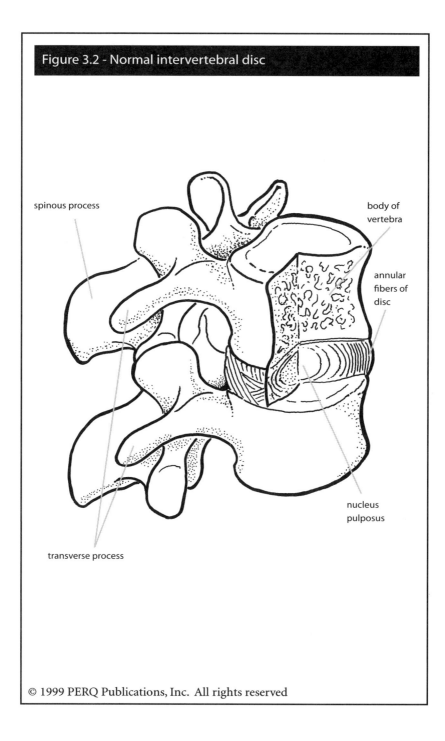

Figure 3.2 - Normal intervertebral disc

spinous process

body of vertebra

annular fibers of disc

nucleus pulposus

transverse process

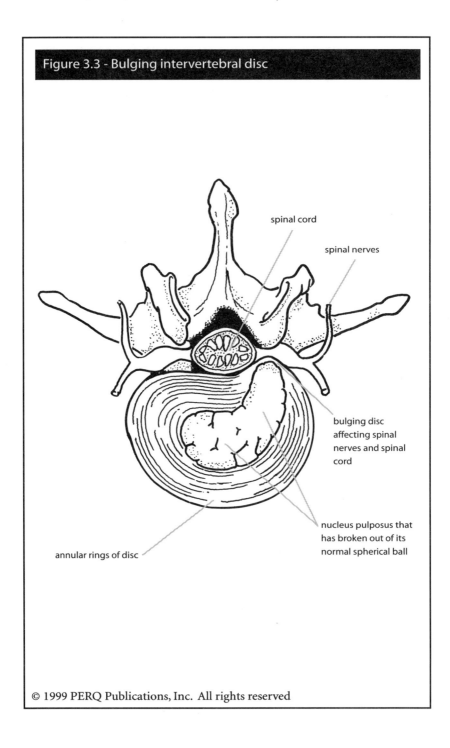

Figure 3.3 - Bulging intervertebral disc

spinal cord

spinal nerves

bulging disc affecting spinal nerves and spinal cord

nucleus pulposus that has broken out of its normal spherical ball

annular rings of disc

lifting causes more microtraumas, or tears, to the surrounding rings, which opens up the possibility that the gelatinous substance inside the ball could spill into the space behind the disc. This is where the real pain begins. I strongly caution my painful low-back patients not to do any lifting, raking, or shoveling—no lifting baskets of laundry or vacuuming, either.

Now, let's get back to Todd. In 1995, Illinois fire fighters started a new health program in which they were expected to run, exercise, lift weights, and then go through a complex obstacle course, set up to simulate experiences they would have while fighting a fire. For instance, they were required to climb up and down ladders; pull themselves up, down, and out of obstructed areas; and pull a 170-pound dummy on a sled while clothed in their heavy fire-proof gear. In a real fire, *none* of these activities would necessarily injure a lower back, but, putting them all together—running an obstacle course of one strenuous activity after another—was too much. Although Todd was young (23 years old at the time), the combination of intense exercises and running caused the disc between Todd's fourth and fifth lumbar vertebrae to spit a piece of the gelatinous substance out toward the spinal canal.

This was the first time Todd had ever experienced any low back problems, and his surgeon expected him to say "yes" and be in surgery that same afternoon or the next day. His mother, however, encouraged him to get a second opinion and to see if a naprapathic chiropractor could help. He walked into my office with an armful of CAT scans, MRIs and X-rays. I was extremely cautious. One good tug or pull might have sent the rest of that disc into the spinal canal, and I didn't want to see that.

Todd also had severe foot drop affecting the ankle of his left foot— a good indication that the nerve is pinched somewhere along its path, which suppresses the ability of the foot to hold its natural position. I applied the naprapathic treatment of gently rocking and coaxing Todd's muscles, ligaments, tendons, and bones in an effort to supply the whole area with blood and let the body be its own

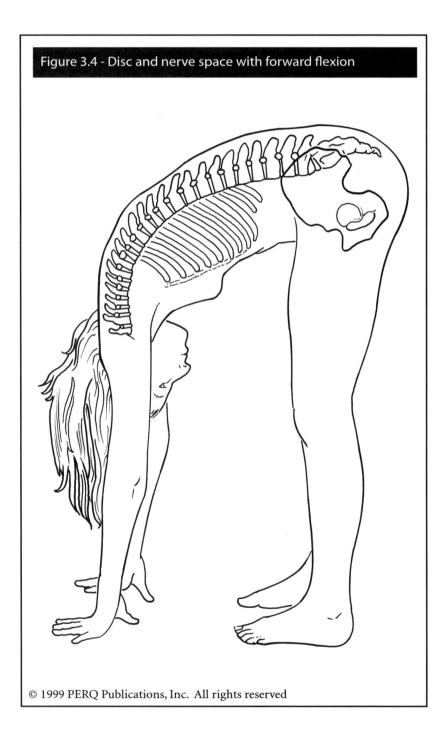

Figure 3.4 - Disc and nerve space with forward flexion

healer. After one such treatment, Todd's pain, which had been radiating down his entire leg, changed its pattern. Although he no
longer had pain in his thigh, he did have pain from his calf to the
bottom of his foot, where he had originally experienced it. We
waited a day and a half and gave him another mild naprapathic
treatment with lots of massage, stretching, and traction in the
lower back.

The third time he came to see me, Todd no longer had any pain in
his foot or ankle. He had one painful spot on the outside, or lateral
side, of his calf and the ability of his foot to flex had greatly
improved. Moreover, there were almost no symptoms in his lower
back, and almost no pain associated with the disc herniation. Two
and a half weeks later, Todd was completely pain free. I have rarely
seen improvement this rapid and dramatic, but Todd was young
and the body is an amazing healer. What the body lays down, the
body can pick back up. If the body extrudes a piece of disc, it can
generate the necessary elements for going in there and picking up
that extruded piece. However, in order for that healing to occur,
Todd's body—all of our bodies—must stop the irritation and take
in the proper nutrients so that the blood can carry them to the
problem area.

Exercises for the Lower Back
Flexion
The primary exercise I recommend to 95 percent of my patients with
low-back injuries, strains, or general low-back stiffness involves bending
forward, or forward flexion. Because it widens the spaces between the
bones, [**Figure 3.4**] forward flexion allows excellent circulation to filter
all the joints and spaces of the lower back. On the other hand, backward bending, or extension, places the bones in the lower spine closer
together, limiting the amount of space the nerves have to exit the
spine. [**Figure 3.5**] These points of exit are called *foramen*, and if
arthritis or calcium deposits have rearranged their normal shape,
extension can entrap a nerve and cause more pain and stiffness.

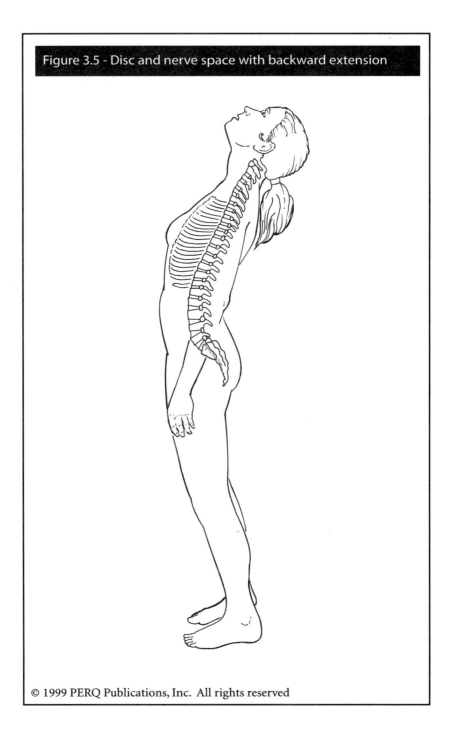

Figure 3.5 - Disc and nerve space with backward extension

The Third-World Squat

I suggest that my patients practice an exercise I call "the third-world squat" on a regular basis. [**Figure 3.6**] This is a marvelous squatting position assumed by native people thereby making chairs unnecessary. We should remember that unlike North Americans, the people of the third world who still retain a diet rich in fish, plant proteins, and fiber from fruits and vegetables suffer a much lower incidence of low-back aches and pains, specifically disc disease. This is primarily because they don't eat large amounts of beef, pork, chicken, or lamb. This helps them avoid the mineral depletion that comes from eating meat.

The third-world squat, done regularly (I suggest morning, noon, and night—more often if possible) stretches and tractions the muscles, tendons, ligaments, and bones in the lower back so that blood, with its proper nourishment, can get into all parts of the spine.

Start by firmly grasping a couch, cabinet or piece of furniture that is heavier than you are. Then attempt to squat, keeping the heels planted squarely on the floor. Spread your knees apart past the side of the body and squat, flexing knees parallel to the chest, or tighten the curve of the upper body so that the stretch is greater for the lower back. Now relax and breathe deeply into the squatting position, and hold the position for one to three minutes.

Within the first 30 seconds, the body responds with a tendon reflex that doesn't allow the muscles to stretch beyond acceptable limits. The tendons at the end of each muscle are saying, "This is going to rip us completely off the bones! Prepare to stop this guy right in his tracks!" You don't get too far when you initially stretch into the squatting position because your tendons shut down and refuse to let you overstretch.

As you begin to breathe, start relaxing into the position. After 30 to 40 seconds, your tendons realize that they are not going to be ripped from their bony attachments and they relax, allowing a greater lengthening stretch of the center of the muscle. This opens

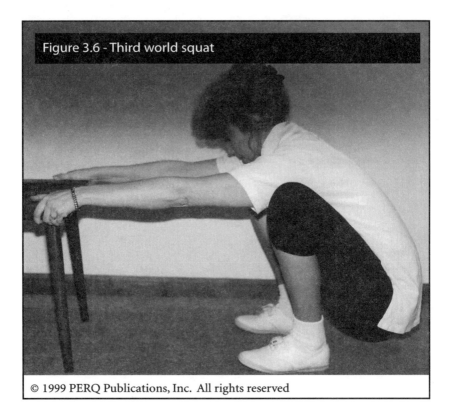

Figure 3.6 - Third world squat

up new avenues for blood to flood in between the fibers. After one minute, you'll find that you can stretch a little further. And as you sustain that stretch to the two-minute and the three-minute mark, you can push it even more.

When finished (two to three minutes of stretching are plenty), rise slowly. There is usually some stiffness, but that is normal, especially if you're over thirty-five. You've had all that blood rushing to your forward-flexed position, so when returning to the standing position, the blood has to rush back to the opposite muscles. After your squat session, use Zheng Gu Shui to recirculate the blood to all areas.

If you are performing this stretch regularly and your stiffness remains unchanged, check your calcium-mineral levels. Raise the calcium levels for a few days and see if some of the stiffness disappears. Are you eating dark-green leafy foods? Are you taking calcium-mineral supplements with coffee? Remember, coffee prevents you from absorbing the calcium, so take it in the evening when you go to bed. Are you eating too much beef or drinking carbonated beverages? Both of these substances steal your calcium. I advise my patients that stiffness in the muscular system is not a disease. It is a *communication system* used by our bodies to let us know that we are low on nutrients. Add the calcium and the stiffness usually disappears.

It's difficult to generalize for every single patient, but this squat will often deliver nutritious blood, stretch the soft tissue and help heal the lower back. Occasionally, a patient walks in with built-up scar tissue surrounding the spine, calcium deposits on the spine, or injury to an area where bone alignment malformation has occurred. Your body will tell you what feels good and what doesn't. Do the squat a couple of times. After the initial tightness, is the exercise getting easier? Observe whether the lower back has less tension during the day. Are episodes of tension less frequent or for a shorter duration? Is your pain level reduced? Learning to understand your body's language means shutting off the radio and television and being *with* your body during your periods of exercise. Minute observations are important when learning to understand your body's communication.

Side Bends

After the back is stabilized and pain free, another exercise I recommend is side bends.[**Figure 3.7**] I like this routine because it tightens all the muscles around the entire waist from the back to the front. Side bends, while trimming the waist, also strengthen the front stomach musculature, which takes the strain off the back paraspinal muscles (the muscles along both sides of the spine). Besides, I can't seem to get myself on the floor to do sit-ups because they are so tough to do. Exhausted after only 15 crunching-type sit-ups, my motivation just slips away, so I concentrate on side bends instead.

Stand erect, with knees bent slightly forward. Bend forward a little at the waist—just enough to take the backward arch out of the lower back. Raise your hands over your head and clasp them together. Slowly—very slowly—bend to the side. The more slowly you bend, the more muscle fibers will be involved. Bend to the side as far as you can and then return to the upright position—again as slowly as possible.

Start with five repetitions on each side, morning and evening, for a day or two. Increase the repetitions by five, every third day, until you reach thirty repetitions on each side, two or even three times per day. Around the second or third day, the sides of your mid-abdominal area will feel like someone kicked you. These muscles, tucked under the ribs, are never used in such normal everyday activities as doing laundry, cutting the grass, or walking the dog, so after just a few of these wonderful waist-slimming bends, they may be screaming in pain.

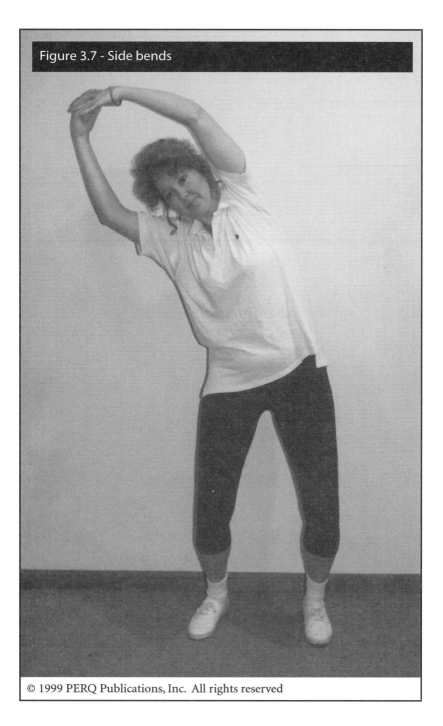

Figure 3.7 - Side bends

Chapter 4

Neck Care

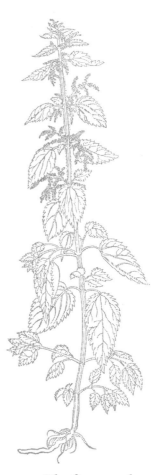

Neck

The neck is a complicated piece of equipment. The first vertebra is shaped like a ring. The second is a pin-like structure that sticks up into that ring. [**Figure 4.1**] Together, the two vertebrae allow our head to pivot around the center axis of the second vertebra, giving us the ability to turn our heads to the right and left a possible 45 degrees in each direction. The rest of the vertebrae of the neck slide forward and backward in a gliding motion, giving us the ability to bend our necks forward and backwards. The ligaments between each bone and the bony eminences on the vertebrae limit our ability to flex forward or bend backward in the neck. The way each bone of the neck sits on another creates a natural convex curve similar to the convex curve of the lower back. We acquire the neck curve at the age of three months when we develop the muscle strength to hold our heads up. We acquire the lumbar curve at the base of the spine when we develop the strength to stand and walk. Thus, each curve is created as our bodies mature.

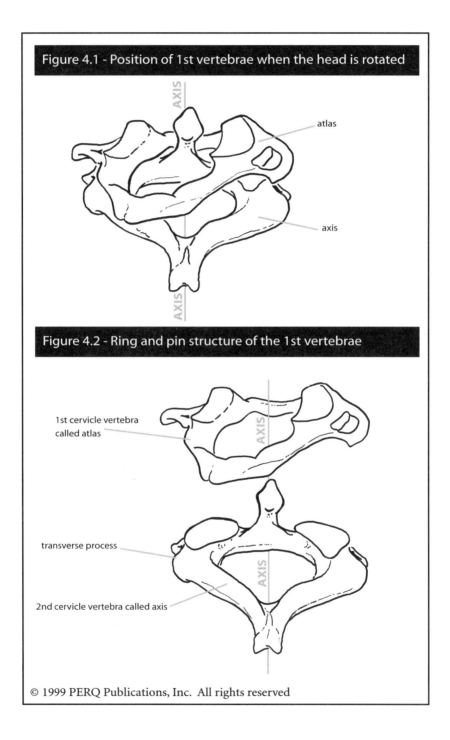

Figure 4.1 - Position of 1st vertebrae when the head is rotated

atlas

axis

Figure 4.2 - Ring and pin structure of the 1st vertebrae

1st cervicle vertebra called atlas

transverse process

2nd cervicle vertebra called axis

Our bodies also have two opposite concave curves. One is in the center of the back parallel with the heart, and the other one forms the curve of our buttocks at the bottom of the spine, where the sacrum and the coccyx bones have been fused together. These two sets of parallel curves in the body are held in place by the position of each bone and the strength of the supporting soft tissue, tendon, muscle, and ligament. The dictionary describes tension as mental, emotional, or nervous strain, the physical results of which are muscle spasms that can cut off circulation and alter normal nerve flow. Tension held in the neck and shoulders (which we feel in our necks as tightness or stiffness) can distort the shape of the normal spinal curve. Tension held in the shoulders can put strain on all the muscles that run up to the head. These muscles also lift the scapulae, or the wing bones in the upper back, and the shoulders. When they spasm, tension is created in the neck, which can affect the way we carry our heads.

Unlike the ball and socket joints found in the hips and upper arms, the head is a heavy round ball with no bony support—it has only the strength of the ligaments and muscles to hold it up. In proper alignment, these soft tissues finger down into the bones of the shoulders and support the head. In my practice, I have lifted quite a few heads—some extremely heavy. For two years, my office was located in a health club and some of my patients were very large weight lifters. But whether I'm dealing with everyday tension, a sports injury to the neck, or the effects of an automobile injury to the head, taking the head's weight off the neck lets blood rush into the cellular spaces, joints, and muscle fibers.

To work on necks, I place patients on their backs, with their heads resting on a support piece on my treatment table. This head-support piece allows me to slip my hands underneath the neck and to massage the musculature that lies on each side of the spine. I then use manual traction in which I cradle the head in my hands at the base of the skull, and gently pull the head away from the body for two or three minutes. Next, I test each cervical vertebra, (each of the seven spinal bones in the neck is referred to as a cervical vertebra). They each have

two bony wings (one on each side) called the transverse processes.
[**See Figures 4.1 and 4.2**]

As a naprapathic-chiropractic physician, I test for soreness, deep
pain, and position by feeling through the many muscle layers of
the neck to find these transverse processes. I then exert a small but
even amount of pressure on each and question the patient as to pain
levels. Pain on one side or the other means buckled fibers and is
an indication that those fibers are not the ones I want to push on.
In other words, the patient's pain tells me what not to do. Pain is
just another method of communication our bodies have developed
to help us function at optimal levels.

As I connect with the transverse processes, I get an immediate feel
for the position of each vertebra. Individual vertebra can rotate
so that one transverse process (on the right side, for example)
appears to be toward the back of the body, while the process on
the left is rotated toward the front of the body. This torque can
affect just one bone or can twist the entire neck. The result of this
rearrangement of the normal cervical curve can be an achy neck,
sore shoulders, numb or tingling arms or fingers, headaches, or
even an upset stomach when that torque is great enough to involve
muscles and nerves.

These problems can also be made worse if the normal cervical curve
is not reinforced on a daily basis. We spend a great deal of the day
looking down—chopping vegetables, working at our computers,
talking to the kids, or eating a meal. Sixty or seventy years of bending
forward like this and our necks are permanently fused in this position. Lying flat on our backs and getting shoulders that have been
slumped forward all day into their normal position, helps return the
neck to its correct curve. While we sleep, we need to keep our necks
in their original curve by placing some kind of support underneath. This allows our bones, muscles, ligaments, nerves, and the entire
neck to rest.

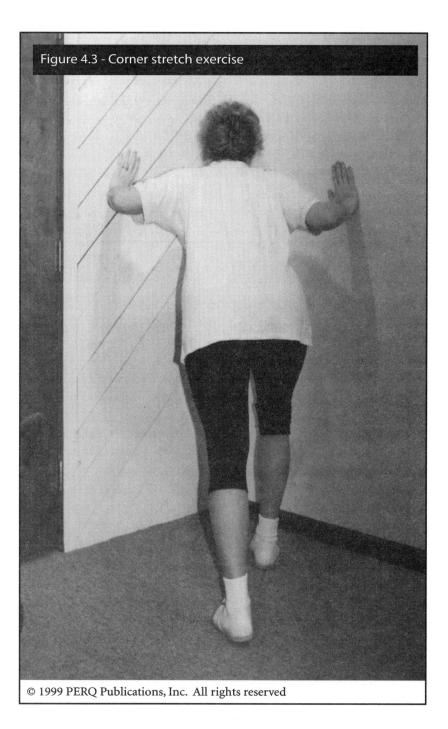

Figure 4.3 - Corner stretch exercise

If you've been sleeping on several pillows for years, your neck has molded itself into the head-forward pose; thus, a flat-on-your-back position may be quite uncomfortable at first. Start with a cervical roll under one pillow for a week of two while you do exercises [**See Figure 6.2 - the "Corner Stretch" exercise pictured here and explained in detail on pages 107-08**] to stretch out the muscles in the front of the chest that hold the shoulders forward and the head bent down.

You can also try a bath towel that has been rolled to a thickness of about three to four inches. Lie flat on your back and place the rolled towel under the back of the neck. Even if you spend most of the night on your side, keep the towel in place. The objective is to feel the support without feeling like there is a hard lump under your neck. If it feels like a rock, the towel is too thick. I give my patients a foam roll, approximately three inches thick, that can be used alone or put into the pillow case where the neck meets the pillow.

I insist that my patients start their evening's rest lying on their backs with their heads and shoulders flat on the bed, rolled towel under the neck. *No pillow at all!* Orthopedic pillows with the centers hollowed out are a good way to support the natural cervical curve, but even these pillows slightly raise the head up from the absolutely flat plane of the bed. This gives the body at least ten to fifteen minutes to stretch back into its upright position after a day bent forward.

More Blood, Please

Simple neck stiffness, the inability to turn one's head, frozen shoulders and even headaches all require increased circulation. The primary objective is to use massage to pump nutrient-rich blood to the neck, shoulders, and the base of the head.

Start by looking in your refrigerator (where all your cooking oils should be) for sweet almond, peanut, or olive oil. All nut oils work great for sore, tight, achy muscles. Always pour the oil into your palm first to warm it—cold oil straight out of a bottle tends to shock the patient. And avoid massaging the hard parts of the bones—the part that sticks out, that hurts. I always concentrate on these areas when I'm trying to generate circulation to a patient's upper body.

Vary the kind of strokes you use. Applying the same stroke on the same area for a couple of minutes can cause patients to feel as though you're digging a hole in their skin. Try round circular motions for 30 seconds then switch to long strokes that run in the direction of the muscle's length. Allow your thumbs to use long fluid strokes, and then switch to small circles with your fingertips. Next, switch to a stroke using the edge of the palm on the side where the little finger is. A variety of strokes allows you to use a variety of your own muscles. This prevents hand fatigue and lets you massage longer and do a more thorough job.

I stand over my patients, which allows me to use my upper-body weight with my arms outstretched—in effect, leaning on the patient without using much muscle strength at all. If you're working on a bed, put your patient close to the edge and stand over them. Or try using a couch. After massaging the side of the body that is *farther* away from you for ten minutes, have the patient change positions (move the feet to where the head was).

Surprised that I said "farther away?" Placing your fingers about one-half inch away from the spine on the opposite side of the body from where you're standing, and firmly sliding your hands over the paraspinals toward the outside of the body, is a wonderful technique for promoting spinal circulation and can only be done from the opposite side of the body.

Remember that if you're the patient, you know where it hurts and you must communicate this. You know what fibers are involved. Do not be afraid to tell your spouse, partner or massage therapist what feels good and what does not. Find the center of the pain. Is it a toothache-like pain? Start massaging around this area first, and move the largest joint close to it to drain the excess fluids. The swelling is composed of the body's healing soldier cells carrying away the fluids and inflammation that your body builds in and around the painful site. In order for new blood to carry in additional healing elements, the old debris must leave. This is one important function of massage and allows the body to heal much faster.

A massage usually feels good; but often, with a medicinal massage, some areas are going to hurt. Start by taking it easy. As the new influx of blood penetrates the problem area, the pain lessens. This happens most often when the problem is a muscle, ligament, tendon or nerve. Although massage is a key component on the road to health with joint pain, you may not see relief at the time of the first massage. Red pepper, black pepper, and chili peppers set joints on fire. Your massage will do nothing until those items are removed from the diet.

Start a massage at the heart—where our energy originates—even if the problem is in the wrist. Blood flows from the heart, so it is at the heart that I or you must begin pushing fresh blood to the problem area. All of this is done on the patient's back. Begin with the large muscles, called the paraspinals, that lie on each side of the spine. Start one-half inch away from the bones that protrude in the spine and take care not to massage any closer to the spine. We call that half inch on either side of the spine the "uncomfortable zone."

Although the heart area is between the spine and the scapula, or wing bone, on the left side of the body, both sides of the upper back must be massaged in order to keep the body balanced. The energy of the heart actually affects both the right and left sides of the paraspinal muscles. I have found that when one side of the middle of the back feels more painful or sensitive to the touch, the opposite side holds more tension and feels more dense (some folks' muscles feel more like rocks than soft body tissue). Use small circular motions and long, slow, pulling motions along the length of the muscle groups. And if your fingernails are short enough, use fingertip circles, without moving your hands.

This brings me to a very important point about nails and the shape of the fingers. Some people are born with fingernails that, even when kept short, extend past the ends of their fingertips. These kinds of nails are difficult to keep out of the way. When these folks perform medicinal massages on themselves, they need to carefully observe what feels good and what hurts. When massaging someone else, they need to ask for feedback and be receptive to using more of the fleshy part of the thumbs. If they use the edges of their thumbs, they may unknowingly dig a nail into the patient's skin.

I am short of stature and the pads of my fingers extend past the length of my fingernails. Thus, my nails appear to be very short. I now know that I was born with these puffy little pads for the specific purpose of doing body work. I can get in deep and feel those muscles and the bones in the neck with an incredible sensitivity. My hands help me listen to what my patients' body structures are saying, and I thank the Great Spirit for them. But I hope that in my next lifetime I get long, elegant fingernails!

Once you have massaged the center of the back, the shoulders, and the tops, sides, and backs of the arms where they join the back, move toward the troubled area, if you haven't already arrived at that point. Follow our rule of staying about a half inch from the midline of the spine when massaging up the neck. The face can be supported by two pillows under each cheek, with a space in the center for the nose to breathe, but keep the pillows low so that the neck is not arched too much. I usually seat myself at the top of my patient's head and use both thumbs simultaneously to massage the paraspinal musculature in the neck.

After massaging the paraspinals, have your patient flip over on his back on the floor while you sit above his head with your legs out in a V-shape. Cup both hands under the neck, with thumbs off to the side not touching the neck. Gently traction the head by pulling it toward you at the point where the neck and head join, using enough pull so that your partner says it feels good. This is manual traction. With children, use less pull and also ask for their feedback.

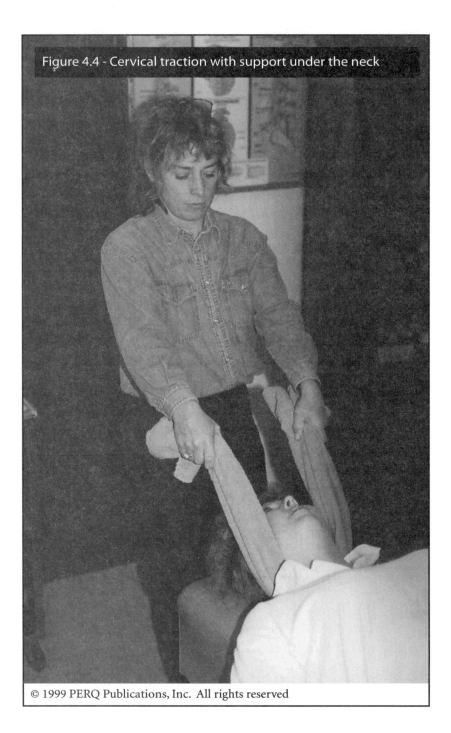

Figure 4.4 - Cervical traction with support under the neck

There is another simple and easy manual traction technique that you can do at home with your partner. Roll an ordinary bath towel lengthwise into a long thin roll—a thick, luxurious towel can be too bulky to handle. Have your partner lie on his back and place the towel behind his neck so that it cradles his skull. Hold both ends of the towel and lean back so that the towel pulls slightly up and backward in a diagonal direction. [**Figure 4.4**]

Begin with light traction—using just enough tension so that the patient is comfortable, but not so much as to move him, and do not put any pressure on the ears or jaws. This traction can be held for two to four minutes.

Because children are flexible, buoyant, and lively, and because they recover from injury so quickly, they are less likely to need any kind of neck traction. However, this neck-traction technique can be part of a treatment for lymphatic drainage of the head when ear infections, cold and sinus problems or flu symptoms are present. It will help move the child's congestion from in front of the sinuses and under the ear canals back into the body. Once there, the congestion can be broken down into a less toxic form and excreted through the liver and intestines. Manual traction delivers nourishing blood to the muscles of the neck and shoulders, and also pulls the bones of the neck apart and saturates the inner joints, ligaments and protective covering of the spinal cord with fresh blood. Rubbing or brushing the scalp continues the flow of blood toward the brain.

Check with your local library or health food store for books on massage techniques. Practice on friends and loved ones. Ask for feedback with each session and note what hurts and what feels good. Regular massage or naprapathic treatments are your most inexpensive good-health insurance. Massaging the shoulders and neck, and naprapathic alignment of each vertebra in the neck and upper back, ensure that nutrients reach the innermost tissues of the neck and back.

A problem with muscle tension, bone alignment, circulation, and nerve flow through the neck and shoulders can cause problems in the arms and hands, often experienced as numbness or tingling. Blood and nerves must travel through these regions before descending to the upper arms, elbows, forearms, and hands. Stiffness, tightness, and loss of full range of motion to the neck and shoulders can prevent full transmission of both blood and nerve impulses down to the extremities. I use a combination of Chinese theory about the strength of the heart, Chinese herbs, American vitamins, and a good naprapathic treatment to get these natural tools where I want them to go.

All blood and energy flows from the heart, so our therapy must concentrate on the heart first. If the body's vital energy is not strong, the body will conserve what vitality exists for the heart first. Circulation to the extremities is of secondary importance when the heart is the body's primary concern. We have a brilliant system that automatically shuts down unnecessary circuits when the main power center is under attack—space-age battle tactics in a body designed thousands of years ago.

Dr. Lisa Lau explains that Chinese medical theory looks to the strength of the heart when examining insufficiencies in the arms and hands. Diets high in dense animal foods, such as beef, pork, lamb, and butter, steal the heart's energy—as do nerve-depleting foods, such as coffee, alcohol, white sugar, flour, and cold drinks. The calcium and mineral loss from the heavy proteins found in animal foods cause muscle spasms in the chest, shoulders, and neck. These spasms pull bones out of perfect alignment which, in turn, cause the nerves exiting these bones to be cramped and twisted. The result is altered nerve signals up and down their fibers. That's why our hands become numb at night or start tingling every time we use our fingers to do tight, concentrated work like sewing or writing. Just picking up that coffee cup (filled, of course, with hot herbal tea) is difficult. Other symptoms can include an unexplained painful elbow or carpal tunnel syndrome. Adding calcium for muscles and B-complex for nerve transmission will help, but for the best results, always take the whole B-complex, not individual B vitamins. These vitamins exist in nature as a whole complex. Mother Nature does not grow B6 on trees.

Before rushing off to the cardiac surgeon for an EKG or a stress test, consider why your heart is weak. Weakness of the heart begins long before you're wheeled in for your first triple bypass. This kind of sickness comes from being in the wrong job, unable to achieve your life's passion. Working long hours, day after day, can also steal the heart's strength. Or, it can be the result of remaining in a relationship where the love has been taken over by anger and ego-sustaining righteousness. Addressing these issues lessens stress factors that create physical illness and reinforces the belief that the *wholeness* in holistic healing isn't confined to muscle, bone, and blood. Take time to be with your *self* and ask yourself the real cause of your health patterns. You hold the answers somewhere inside of you.

Massage techniques for headaches are similar to those used to relieve stiffness to the neck, shoulders, and base of the head. Headache massage incorporates three important points that open circulation to the entire head, so be sure to read the next section even if you don't experience this particular problem.

Chapter 5

Help for Headaches

Headaches

Because headaches are induced by different things, we must find the cause before we can properly treat them. Questions and answers are an important part of this procedure: Where is your headache located? Is it in the front or the back of the head? Different headaches occur at different times of the day. Are your headaches morning headaches or after-work headaches? Do they occur when you're tired from hard physical labor that uses lots of muscle energy? These headaches are different from those occurring after eating certain foods or not eating anything at all for hours on end. I require my patients to keep a detailed log of what they've eaten for a week or a month to more accurately analyze their pain.

Back-of-the-Head Headaches

First, let's explore the headache that occurs at the back of the head and neck. Does it occur regularly, for instance—one to two times a week or one to two times a month? Does it have a repeating pattern of occurrence? With pain at the back of the head or neck,

I usually suspect that calcium requirements are not being met. We have a lot of muscular tissue back there that holds the head on top of the neck. The head is held in place by many layers of paraspinal muscles and ligaments that reach down from the skull and attach to each vertebra and the scapulae, commonly referred to as the wing bones of the back. [**Figure 5.1**]

These muscles are under constant strain due to the changing position of the head during the day, especially when we look down. We spend our waking hours performing a hundred tasks with our heads and necks bent down. That position continually stresses these muscles. Every time a muscle moves or contracts, our bodies move calcium and magnesium in and out of the cellular spaces that surround that muscle. The mineral requirements are very high for these muscles because they hold the neck in a bent position most of the time.

If these muscles don't have enough minerals, chiefly calcium and magnesium, they don't go flaccid and fail to work. They spasm instead. They go into overtime, tighten, and don't let go. As a result, we feel tension in the neck. If we move that neck and say, "Boy, is my neck stiff!" it means the neck is in a spasm and needs more calcium and magnesium.

Calcium is the predominant mineral in the body. The daily calcium requirements set by the National Research Council are approximately 800 milligrams per day. Most calcium supplements available at the local health food store automatically mix calcium with magnesium in a ratio of 2-to-1. When I recommend 1200 to 1500 milligrams of calcium for a neck experiencing tight spasms, I assume that the magnesium levels are about 600 to 750 milligrams. Green foods have this perfect balance of calcium to magnesium. Too much calcium can cause constipation, but during a headache, calcium concentrations are usually very low in our systems.

When a patient is experiencing a headache, I recommend starting with 1200 milligrams and then adding an extra 500 milligrams

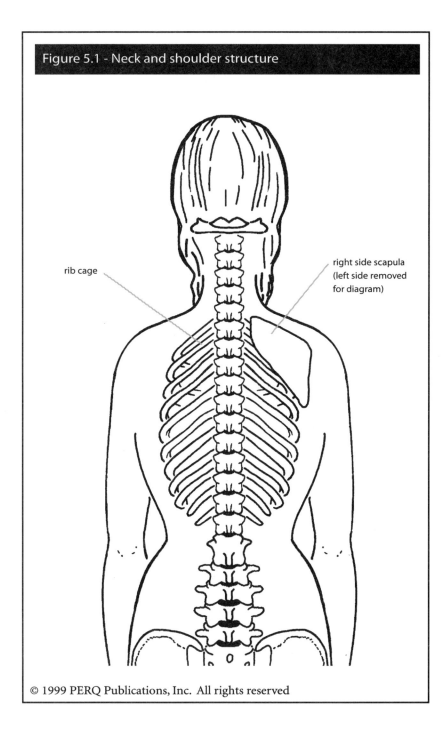

Figure 5.1 - Neck and shoulder structure

rib cage

right side scapula
(left side removed
for diagram)

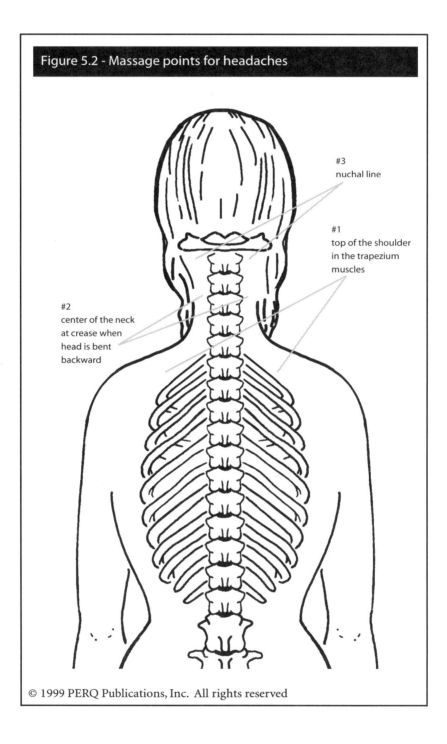

Figure 5.2 - Massage points for headaches

#3
nuchal line

#1
top of the shoulder
in the trapezium
muscles

#2
center of the neck
at crease when
head is bent
backward

approximately every two to three hours during the course of the headache, until a maximum of 2000 to 2500 mg is reached within a 24-hour period. I understand that's a lot of calcium, but if you are experiencing a neck spasm, you can never have enough. I do not recommend a dose this large on a daily basis without first performing a comprehensive examination of the patient and studying all the variables of his or her unique situation.

With almost every headache, the neck muscles are so tense that they squeeze the blood vessels, often inhibiting circulation to the brain. Of course, some blood does get to the brain, but it does not exit the head as efficiently as it enters. We end up with a surplus of blood that actually squeezes the brain and causes tension headaches.

Once calcium levels have been raised, the second half of the treatment ensures that the mineral-rich blood gets to the tight neck. Neck tension is often so pronounced that good circulation is almost impossible without a little help from soft-tissue massage, or naprapathic massage, at three primary points.

The first is toward the top of the shoulders in the trapezium muscles, on both the right and left sides. [**Figure 5.2**] While massaging, pay attention to the more painful side. Although you can do it yourself, it can be more effective to let someone help you.

The second point lies in the neck, halfway between the head and the shoulders at the point where the neck seems to crease the most when the head is bent backward. This massage, which you can perform on yourself, is done with the ends of the third finger. Use the left hand to manipulate the left side of the neck and the right hand for the right—about a fingertip's width away from the bones of the spine. While your head is bent backward, press in deeply and massage the deep muscles in the neck.

The third important point is along the nuchal line. This line separates the neck from the head and, as my boyfriend pointed out, "is way too high to still be part of the neck." This nuchal line, or base of the skull, is the point where energy from the lower body intersects with energy from the head. Headaches are caused by the inability of the two energy flows to integrate. With your thumb, massage in small circular motions, moving across the line from one side to the other. Is one side more sore than the other? Is the pain like a toothache? Is it almost too sore to touch? This is the side you want to massage twice as much as the other.

These three points should be manipulated about 20 minutes after taking the calcium-mineral supplement. It takes about that long for the minerals to break down and circulate through the blood stream. Although you can begin massaging as soon as your headache symptoms appear, you should repeat the process again, 20 minutes after taking the supplement.

I also suggest rubbing the neck and shoulders with a product called Rescue Remedy cream, which is commonly found in your local health food store. In liquid form, Rescue Remedy is made from five different flowers that have been picked at full sunlight when the plant's energy is up in the petals. The petals are put into distilled water for a few hours and then discarded. What remains is the distilled water mixed with only the flower's essence. Not even a molecule of the flower is present—just its essence. The essence is so small it can enter through a cell's protective outer wall without resistance because it needs no cellular transport.

The homeopathic principle here is similar to the principle of immunization. With immunization, an injection of the infectious organism is introduced into the bloodstream so that the body will begin creating a defense mechanism to fight invasion of even larger doses of the infectious agent. The homeopathic remedy, which is made from animal, vegetable, or mineral sources, is made into a very small dilution. If the animal, mineral, or vegetable source were taken at a very large dose, it would produce in a healthy person symptoms similar to those of the disease. The fundamental law upon which homeopathy is based is the law of similars or "like is cured by like"—in Latin, *Similia similibus curentur*. Hippocrates wrote in 400

B.C. that "Through the like, disease is produced, and through the application of the like, it is cured." The law of similars states that the very small dose of a remedy can cure a disease if it produces symptoms in a healthy person similar to those of the disease, in this case our headache symptoms[1]. The correct remedy kicks the cell into gear toward normalcy because it is a very minute dose of what, at a much larger dose, would cause the same symptoms.

Rescue Remedy is recommended anytime a cell needs rescuing from trauma, emotional distress, headaches, upset stomach, etc. I once used Rescue Remedy with a patient who had gone into shock. He separated his shoulder when a horse he'd been holding suddenly reared up. He grabbed his shoulder, collapsed to the ground, and began to get pale, sweat profusely, and to lose consciousness. One dropper, administered sublingually (i.e., under the tongue), and within 30 seconds he was back to full consciousness and regaining his color.

The manufacturer also dissolves this remedy into a cream that comes in a tube. You can squeeze out approximately one and a half inches of the cream and rub it on the back of the neck and on the shoulders to alleviate headaches. I recommend rubbing in this amount every half hour that the headache continues.

The liquid form of Rescue Remedy is the last important component of therapy for headaches that occur in the neck and back of the head. One dropper can be taken sublingually every three to five minutes for the first twenty minutes of the headache. Then one dropper can be taken every ten to fifteen minutes for the next two or three hours. If the headache still persists after that time, continue to take the Rescue Remedy, but further examination of mineral levels and of outside influences also must be made. Such things as your diet during the past twelve hours, toxic smells, and any chemicals that may have come in contact with your skin, including hand and body lotions or cleaning products, must be considered as poisonous components of your headache.

Rescue Remedy is such a subtle therapy that many factors will affect its potency. Touching the glass medicine dropper with your hands, tongue, or sides of your mouth will weaken its potency. This can be avoided by opening your mouth wide, raising your tongue toward the roof of your mouth, tilting your head back, and dropping the liquid into your mouth without allowing the dropper to touch anything. Because of this power to inactivate the treatment, coffee should never be taken near the time that you are using Rescue Remedy, nor should menthol and camphor products, including Zheng Gu Shui or minty-tasting toothpastes, be used at the same time. Menthol and camphor, like caffeine, will inactivate this vibrational remedy.

So, let us recap our recommendations for back-of-the-head headaches. Add calcium minerals immediately. Massage the nuchal line, the back of the neck, and the points on the top of the shoulders to unlock the energy and get your calcium minerals to the muscles. (You can use Rescue Remedy cream, or olive or peanut oil, for this massage.) And, you want to take the liquid form of Rescue Remedy sublingually.

Front-of-the-Head Headaches

When we get headaches in the front of the head, the first thing to suspect is a sensitivity to sugar, artificial sugar products, chemical food additives, colors, dyes, or processed foods. Occasionally, headaches also occur because no food has been eaten for too long a period or because of a general category I term "poisoned blood."

Artificial food products are foods that no longer resemble real foods. They arrive at the grocery store with interesting but confusing terms attached to what used to be whole foods such as processed cheese, low-fat salad dressing, artificial bacon crumbs, and non-dairy whipping cream. Incorporating these kinds of foods regularly in your diet may be a potential source of problem foods that can cause headaches. They are not real food and must be completely eliminated from any healthy person's diet! The only problem with this grandiose statement is that many artificial food products, preservatives, and chemicals are hidden in the everyday foods we eat. So, put on those glasses and carefully read the labels on the food you're eating.

If you get a headache over the eyes, in the forehead or toward the top of the head, make a list of the foods you've eaten within two hours of the onset of the headache, as well as the foods you've eaten the night before. You should pay attention to sugar, chocolate, bananas, turkey, artificial sugar substitutes, caffeine, artificial dyes, colors, preservatives, additives, and regular and diet soda pop. Artificial sweeteners and phosphorous in carbonated drinks will cause the body to excrete calcium, just when you need this mineral to alleviate the neck tension or muscle spasms making the headache worse. Moreover, not only will carbonated drinks steal calcium from the muscles' intercellular spaces, they can also rob your supply of calcium from bone reserves, which leads to osteoporosis.

Keep a written log of everything you've eaten for the last week and continue it for another week after the onset of the headache. And, don't take this suggestion lightly. Most folks try to keep the list in their heads, and in the process, forget to record a whole food here and an "innocent" slightly processed food there. Of course, they continue to have headaches until I rope them to a chair, stick a pen in their hands, and insist on a list of everything they've eaten the day before the headache. And guess what? It always becomes apparent what's causing their headaches. One patient found bananas were the problem, and another discovered it was turkey. Neither of them suspected those foods at all.

Sometimes, ridding ourselves of the offending food is easy and sometimes it is not. Unfortunately, we are often addicted to the foods that cause our health problems. Understanding the yin/yang food chart found on page 97 will help you create a balance that excludes the foods that make you sick. Nonetheless, whether or not you recognize the offender, the first thing to do is to reach for that bottle of calcium minerals to calm the tight muscle spasms that are restricting optimal circulation to your head.

The brain has its own barrier against poisons, but with a frontal headache, you might suspect that your barrier has allowed toxic elements to seep into the brain, causing intense pain. Diluting the poisons will help the kidneys flush them out, but it is important *not* to do this flushing with *cold water*. Cold weakens nerves, and yours are already crying out in pain. Instead, use a warm blood-cleansing tea, such as Jason Winters tea, and lots of it. Jason Winters has three herbal blood cleansers: red clover from England, sage from India, and another powerful, unnamed ingredient from China. Because poisons are removed from the blood, incredible amounts of energy are released. I drink four to eight cups of Jason Winters tea a day to sustain the energy I need to do naprapathic-chiropractic treatments—so I don't have to depend on caffeine found in regular or decaffeinated coffee. Don't be fooled into thinking it is caffeine-free unless it says "CAFFEINE FREE." Black tea, some herbal teas (green tea) or simply "tea" also contain caffeine. Read the label or ask at the local health food store for a health practitioner who knows. The folks behind the counter at the health food store do a great job, but unless they have a degree in nutrition, they are not health professionals.

Our blood is like the oil in cars. If the oil is cleaned regularly, the car will run trouble free and have a much longer life. Blood-cleansing teas ensure that our systems run more smoothly and efficiently, so we won't be bogged down with toxins transported by the blood to accumulate in the liver, colon and brain.

The massage points for front-of-the-head headaches are the same three points as for back-of-the-head pain—the shoulders, the neck, and the nuchal line. Massaging can be done with Rescue Remedy, peanut oil, or olive oil. And, as before, Rescue Remedy can also be taken sublingually.

Female-Cycle Headaches

Some headaches occur during the week of, before, or just after a woman's menstrual period. Other headaches occur during ovulation—

the time midway through the menstrual cycle when the ovary releases an egg. These headaches are categorized as hormonal and need special consideration. That special consideration is Women's Precious formula, a two-thousand-year-old Chinese herbal formula containing angelica pubescent, panas ginseng, don quai, angelica sinuses, and saliva miltiorrhiza (see pages 100-104 for a detailed description of these herbs).

When I started working with a traditional Chinese herbalist, I gave my patients bundles of raw herbs, which they were to boil until the original five cups of water cooked down into one cup of concentrated tea. Then they were to drink the single cup each morning while the tea was still hot. These Oriental herbal combinations have incredible healing potential but usually taste *horrible*, so the formula has now been compressed into round pellets that resemble rabbit droppings (and are always good for a laugh the first time a patient sees them).

Oriental practitioners recommend ten pellets of Women's Precious in the morning and ten in the evening, taken with warm water. This regulates the female cycle and alleviates PMS problems, hot flashes, difficulties with menopause, and/or hormonal headaches. If you suffer from hormonal headaches, I suggest that Women's Precious be taken for several months in order to affect a real change. Interestingly enough, brushing the head stimulates the whole female hormonal system. Brushing several times a day with long strokes sends energy to the female centers, and also increases circulation to the head. Massaging the back of the neck, the shoulders, the nuchal line (as previously described), and rubbing the Rescue Remedy cream into these same areas (especially during the hormonal headache), will let the blood flow in and out of the brain.

Most importantly, you must restrict coffee in the diet, and as always with headaches, increase your intake of calcium minerals. Extra calcium supplements, in addition to your approximate 1500 milligram daily dosage, will augment the muscles' tendency to relax and allow blood to flow through the shoulders, neck and brain and back to the head again. During your headache, I recommend an extra 200-400 milligrams every two hours. However, a maximum dose of 2000 to 2500 milligrams is the ceiling for a one-day period. That dose is only recommended to alleviate headaches and should not be taken on an everyday basis. Dark-green leafy foods (both steamed and raw) must also be eaten daily.

Liquid Rescue Remedy is also wonderful for emotional stress, whether during the raging hormones of PMS, or in everyday living. If you have a fight with your spouse or are nervous about an appointment, Rescue Remedy will help you return to a normal emotional state without sedating you. One of my patients took the liquid to her divorce hearing, and put several drops into the water she sipped during the proceedings to help her stay calm, so she would not have to rely on drug therapy. The cream would have worked just as well if she had rubbed it into her hands or the back of her neck.

Rescue Remedy is also a marvelous treatment for children with upset stomachs. Although the liquid is preserved with a very small percentage of alcohol, one or two drops are not enough to bother even the smallest child.

The smaller the concentration, the easier it slips into the cells. So if you want to make the remedy even stronger, you only need to dilute it more. You begin the procedure by diluting the Rescue Remedy in its original bottle. Put seven drops of the original liquid into another clean medicine dropper bottle (one can be purchased from your local pharmacy). Then fill the new bottle with distilled water and shake for several minutes. With this extra-diluted solution of Rescue Remedy, the alcohol content is minuscule. I have patients who are members of Alcoholic Anonymous, and even the smell of alcohol bothers them. So, I make this more diluted solution for them, and it works very nicely.

Because the stomach holds all emotion, emotional distress sometimes manifests itself as an upset stomach, I recommend one dropper of Rescue

Remedy, taken sublingually, every three to five minutes as needed. The liquid also works for stomach distress that comes from overeating, or eating fatty or spicy foods. Take one dropper, and if you still have stomach distress three to five minutes later, take another dropper. Repeat this three to five times until the distress is relieved.

Reflex Points

There are several points on the body that correspond to the health, or reflect the status, of the head. For example, on the hands and feet, both the thumb and first toe (commonly referred to as the "great" toe) correspond to the head and the neck.

Look at your hand. The thumbs of the left and right hands represent, respectively, the left and right side of the neck and head. The pads at the base of each thumb are extremely tender. In these pads are reference points for the thyroid and adrenal glands—the organs that provide a natural barometer of our stress levels and the body's assessment of how we're handling stress. There is also a point on the back of the hand where [**Figure 5.3**] the thumb meets the first finger close to the wrist. Trace all the thumb bones and the bones in the first finger through the palm until you find the point where the two intersect—this point correlates to headache pain. If a headache is felt more strongly in the back of the head on the right side, the more tender point will be on the left hand and vice versa. Massaging this point for two to three minutes helps to open up the circulation to the head, which greatly benefits all types of headaches.

The center of the pad on the underside of the great toe corresponds to the center of the brain; massaging this area improves circulation in and out of the head. During a headache, you might find that both the left and right toes (but often one more than the other) are very painful to the touch or to deep massage. Imagine that the energy the head needs to stay healthy is stuck, causing greater sensitivity in one side more than the other. You should massage both, but concentrate on the more sensitive toe. Massage both sides, the

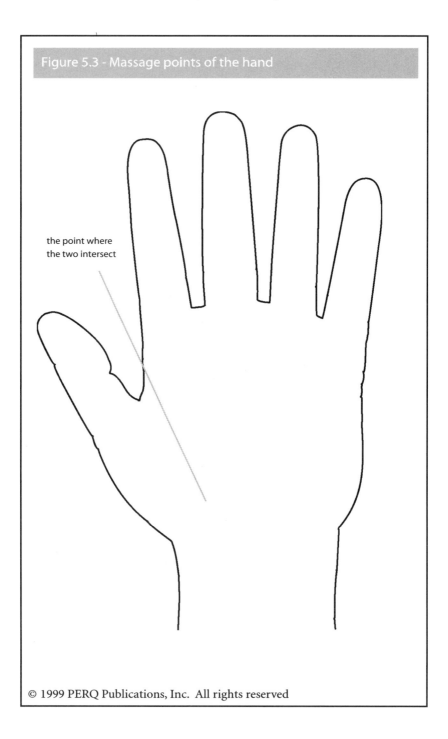

Figure 5.3 - Massage points of the hand

the point where
the two intersect

bottom and the top. Vigorously pull on the toe, stretching it up, down, sideways, and out.

The feet represent many parts of the body [**refer to Figure 3.1 pg 40**]. For example, the existence of athlete's foot may be an indication that there is too much tension around the neck and shoulders because of poor circulation. Massage therapy and naprapathic treatments are needed to open up circulation to the neck. Tightness, achiness, and constant soreness in the toes may be an indication that circulation to the shoulders is poor because they're carrying the weight of the world. In other words, you're taking on too much responsibility and need to lighten the load. The fact that the fungus can survive living on and around the toes can also indicate that the immune system is too overloaded to actively destroy these little freeloaders.

The body communicates in many different ways. I firmly believe that no one just walks into a devastating diagnosis of cancer without previous signs and signals from the body indicating that it was overloaded. Learning the body's communication system may take a lifetime, but the lessons come one disease pattern at a time. We must pay attention to each and every health concern we have.

Now that we've dealt with the physical aspects of headaches and foods that influence them, we need to pay attention to the mental factors. What thoughts were you thinking when you first realized you had a headache? It is important to give yourself permission to no longer have headaches. Say out loud, "I give myself permission to no longer have headaches," and repeat it over and over again. For years your subconscious has been saying, "I have headaches, I get headaches, I've had headaches for years." You've been perpetuating that headache energy. Remember that today is the start of a brand new health attitude—give yourself permission to be healthy.

How Long Does It Take to Get Well?

I can never answer that question. My job is to teach you to be with your body and listen to its responses. With each treatment, you and I reevaluate: Are you feeling better? Are you feeling better for a longer period of time before the pain reoccurs? I can tell you what to look for. Usually after the first treatment, you will find relief in some noticeable form. Is your pain confined to a smaller area? Did your pain get better for an hour—half the day? Could you sleep through the night? Do you feel better two or three days after a treatment, then the pain returns? At that point, or hopefully before that point, someone needs to work on the area again. Naprapathic treatments, massage or gentle massage-like chiropractic adjustments can open the energy that runs to the painful area. But as the energy dwindles, the pain seems to return. So, you should do whatever is necessary to open up that energy, whether it's a treatment, hot compresses, a warm shower, or a Masada bath. This must be done, however, at the time the pain first returns rather than letting it go another week. Without treatment, the original pain levels may return.

You must develop good body awareness and use your health professional's information on maintaining and bringing forth energy to an afflicted area, without signing up for dozens of chiropractic visits. A naprapathic treatment, with its massage-like qualities and light bone movement, is perfect preventative medicine. Because of the physical effort involved in giving naprapathic treatments, I get a treatment every three weeks to keep my energy flowing and to maintain flexibility in my muscles. This keeps me from tightening up or developing areas of stagnated energy, which can breed disease. It is a matter of listening to my own body and developing a timely schedule of maintenance for greater body awareness.

[1.] *Homeopathic Medicine at Home* by Maisimund B. Panos, M.D. and Jane Heimlich, J.P. Tarcher, Inc. Los Angeles 1980, p. 11.

Chapter 6

Easing Nerves, Depression, and Stress

Nerves and Vitamin B-Complex

The nerves are the body's communication pathways. Larger nerves are covered with a myelin sheath that enables nerve transmissions to travel at lightning speeds. The sciatic nerve, the longest nerve in the human body, originates at the bottom of the spine and runs down the back of the leg. When irritated, it can zing pain impulses down the front of the thigh, around the front or back of the knee or to the outside of the calf almost instantaneously as we make the slightest move sideways. [**refer to Figure 2.7 pg 29**] Patients have described nerve pain as an acute pang or as a vague ache, accompanied by numbness or tingling.

Sciatic nerve pain can drop you to your knees and put tears in your eyes, or merely make your lower back stiff and achy. Then again, the pain can be patchy. Tight muscles in the lower back can pinch the sciatic nerve, causing pain to be felt only in the outer side of the calf, skipping the thigh and knee. Eliminating that pain is the patient's number one priority. However, nerves don't often respond independently. When problems arise within the nerves, the holistic practitioner knows that all the surrounding structures play a contributing role in guiding the patient back to normalcy.

It is very difficult to separate bone, muscle, or nerves as the source of the problem. Nerve fibers often run right through the middle of muscle tissue, so once a nerve is irritated, its ability to communicate can develop a few snags. A message from the nerve that would ordinarily tighten a muscle group so that we can take a step forward, instead sends earth-shattering pain signals that prevent us from going anywhere at all. Muscles that spasm from lack of proper nutrition or circulation can squeeze healthy nerve tissue enough to spark pain impulses along the entire course of the nerve. When muscles spasm enough to torque the bones, especially spinal bones, called vertebrae, this also puts tension on the nerve. This is the "ole bone out of place." The muscle is responsible for the bone, which is responsible for the nerves.

Greg points to a spot on the front of his thigh that hurts so badly that it has kept him awake on and off for three weeks. When he sits for any length of time, which he often does at his job, that same pain grabs him as he tries to rise from his chair and makes him look like a man of 95, instead of the 63-year-old youngster that he really is.

Because Greg came into my office specifically for the pain in his leg, he doesn't understand when I start searching the bony points of his lower back for any significant painful point. But his leg is really a large topographical map of regions where the nerves, exiting the lower part of the spine, send their energy. The large sciatic nerve, which is composed of fibers from all the lumbar nerves, branches out to give feeling to each section of the thigh, back of the knee, calf, and foot. If a patient has numbness, tingling or pain wrapping around the front of his groin, I will check the bony protrusion of the third lumbar vertebra for pain or sensitivity. If the pain pattern travels down the front of the thigh to the top of the knee again, I check the third lumbar vertebra. If there's a painful spot on the outside of the calf, I'll check the fourth lumbar vertebra by touching the large bony spinus process at the back of the spine. And I'll ask if it's sore or sensitive on the left or right side. If pain is felt on the top of the foot, I'll check the fifth lumbar vertebra. And just as I expect, Greg's third lumbar spinus process is sensitive on the right side, and it was his right leg that was having all the pain.

We must not forget that nerves go to every part of the body, including the organs. [**Figure 6.1**] When a red, irritated, swollen nerve fiber runs to an organ, the altered transmission can change the organ's ability to operate correctly. Therefore, it is very diffi-cult to tell whether the nerve is the problem or if muscle torquing the nerve, torquing the vertebrae, is the difficulty. Taking a complete history from the patient will give the professional healer good clues with which to evaluate muscle, bone, and nerve symptoms.

Nerve and muscle tissue can't be seen with an X-ray, only bone tissue is visible. But X-raying can harm the bone cells that keep us immune from disease. The only way to really find out what's going on under that skin of ours is to cut ourselves open. Not your favorite option? I wouldn't suggest surgery either, but because muscle tension, bone position, and nerve pathway clearance all need to be addressed, add the optimal nutrition first—B-complex for nerve tissue and calcium and minerals for muscles. I also suggest taking away a few things. Ice-cold foods and drinks, coffee, white sugar, and flour products irritate the myelin sheath that surrounds the nerve, which can make the nerves spark with more pain. With proper nutrition in the blood stream, we are halfway toward allowing the body to be the perfect healing machine it wants to be.

B-complex is the perfect nutrition for nerves, and a good source of it is found in dark-green leafy foods. Mother Nature made these foods the optimal source of digestible minerals such as calcium and magnesium. Therefore we cover both nutritional bases by adding green foods to our diets.

Most of my patients want to add peas and broccoli when I insist that they increase their intake of green food. Peas and broccoli are

Figure 6.1 - Nerves and the organs to which they are related

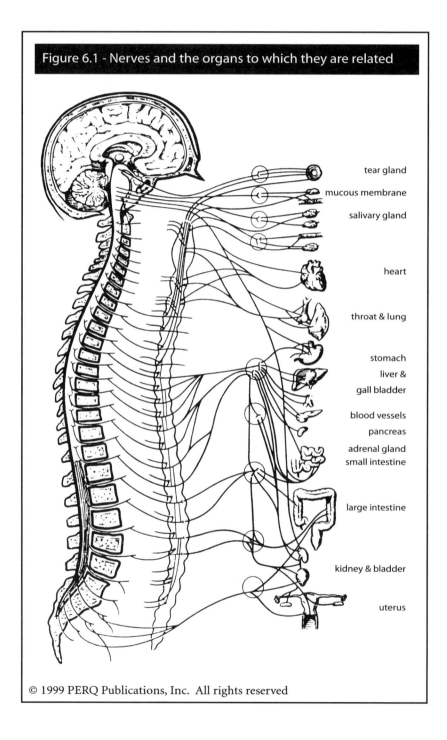

tear gland

mucous membrane

salivary gland

heart

throat & lung

stomach
liver &
gall bladder

blood vessels

pancreas

adrenal gland
small intestine

large intestine

kidney & bladder

uterus

a good start, but what I'm really referring to are *dark-green leafy foods.* Swiss chard, bok choy, romaine lettuce, beet tops, red and green leafy lettuces, and seaweed are not only wonderfully delicious, they are also good, healthy choices. Steaming these leafy greens is the perfect way to cook them. B-complex is a water-soluble vitamin, which means that if it's immersed in water (*e.g.,* when vegetables are boiled), it will leach into the water. You could drink the water, but the objective is to draw the nutrients from the food. (I'm especially fond of picking greens fresh from my garden; in the fall, I either transplant the greens into indoor pots or plant seeds under indoor grow lights.)

I steam the tender young greens for two to four minutes until they have wilted completely, then mix olive oil, unpasteurized apple cider vinegar, and real soy sauce (tamari, composed of soy beans and water), and use this as a light dressing over the greens. (Yes mothers, my twelve-year-old daughter likes these steamed greens, without any coaching from me!) If you are deficient in minerals, your body should relish the taste. But, if you are a finicky eater, you may add your favorite salad dressing.

When life's pace speeds up, and there just isn't time for steamed greens and salad, I often use vitamin supplements. However, since the B vitamins occur in a complete complex in nature, you must not separate them when taking supplements. Ingesting large doses of just B-6, for instance (as a treatment for carpal tunnel syndrome), can knock the other Bs out of kilter.

Complete B-Complex by Rainbow Light is my favorite choice. It's not only a B-complex, but also contains vitamins A and C, bioflavanoids, calcium, magnesium, zinc, potassium, lecithin, barley grass, ginger, hawthorn, Siberian ginseng, bee pollen, and spirulina. This combination of vitamins and herbs enables the body to absorb the B-complex easier and more effectively than some of the other supplements I've tried in my practice. I respect the Rainbow Light name (their multiple vitamin, Nutri-Stars, is the one I choose for my daughter) and suggest that you look for their marvelous Complete B-Complex in your local health food store. Also take a look at some of their other vitamin and herbal combinations. If your store does not carry this line, ask them to order it. It is well worth the time and effort.

White Sugar Substitute

When trying to bring nerves back to a healthy state, white refined sugar is a major detriment. Good whole-food substitutes include honey, fruit concentrates such as chopped raisins or apples, 100 percent maple syrup and date sugar. Date sugar can be found in your local health food store, and is actually roasted dates that have been granulated. It tastes marvelous! My daughter enjoys it sprinkled on oatmeal, cream of rice, and cream of wheat. I use it in my baking and cooking. It will, however, turn baked foods darker than white sugar does.

Two weeks after my patient Karen pulled a hamstring muscle while exercising, she stubbed her toe, which caused a further strain to the back of the thigh where the hamstring muscles are located. Driving put a great amount of pressure on the injury, causing sciatic nerve pains that traveled down to the outside of her calf. But after a few treatments, the injury seemed to be on the mend, with only a slight amount of discomfort occurring when she drove. One day Karen's young daughter insisted on stopping for ice cream. Karen had one scoop of vanilla with strawberries, whipped cream, and pecans! Sounds great, doesn't it? Except that within ten minutes, the discomfort in the back of her hamstring increased to the point where she could hardly drive with her right foot at all! I tell my patients that sugar and cold foods make nerve problems worse. Karen walked into my office later that week exclaiming that she was living proof!

White Bread Substitute

Good substitutes for white bread products are the Manitowoc Natural Ovens breads from Manitowoc, Wisconsin. The company's owner, Paul Stitt, creates the recipes for these breads himself.

Paul has a masters degree in science, and when not in the kitchen, he lectures around the country on foods that make arthritic conditions worse and how whole grains and vegetables can restore good health. Paul combines stone-ground whole wheat flours with oat bran, flax seeds, wheat germ, and extra vitamins and minerals to make some pretty tasty bread. If this bread is not available in your area, be sure to read the entire label on the whole-grain bread in your health food store or grocery. The label must say "whole wheat," not simply "wheat"; otherwise, you may be getting white bread that has been darkened in color instead of a whole-grain product.

Paul's address is:

Natural Ovens of Manitowoc
P.O. Box 730
Manitowoc, WI 54221-0730
Phone 800/772-0730

Coffee Substitute

My favorite hot beverage is Jason Winters Tea, which contains three blood cleansing herbs from around the world—red clover from Europe, sage from India, and an herb from China. It is full of energy and a marvelous substitute for coffee. After four or five hours of physically taxing naprapathic/chiropractic treatments, I drink tea to keep my energy reserves up. A cup every hour increases my energy enough to support the intensive workload needed to maintain my muscles. As with many of my recommendations, you will find this amazing herbal tea only in a health food store.

Imagine that your blood is similar to motor oil that coats each component of your car's engine. If the oil is clean, the car runs more efficiently and has a longer life. The same is true of blood. The cleaner it is, the better your health. Blood-cleansing herbs have the ability to pull toxins out of the blood, leaving you with a cleaner, more efficient system. Your colon and liver are also cleaner and you are less subject to disease. Your body has less garbage to contend with on a daily basis, reducing stress levels throughout your entire body, and promoting longevity.

Jason Winters Tea can be drunk either hot or cool. But, it is important to restate an important Chinese principle: Cold makes nerves weak. During periods of nerve pain, head trauma, and headaches, cold food and drinks will only make the pain worse. I recommend a warm cup of the tea first thing in the morning to break up the congestion in a stuffy head, whether the congestion stems from sinus problems, cold, or flu. I also suggest a warm cup or two for digestive distress or diverticulitis. In her book *Heal Your Body,* Louise Hay attributes dread and the fear of anything new (or the inability to assimilate the new) to stomach and digestive disturbances.[1] Emotional distress can create the opportunity for digestive problems (the stomach is thought to hold all emotions), and many diseases begin with incomplete digestion. Almost all of these unhealthy conditions could benefit from this combination of the three blood cleansers. Besides, Jason Winters Tea is quite flavorful, and the energy it provides the system is caffeine-free.

Caffeine attaches to those precious B-complex vitamins so that they cannot help calm and nourish the nerves. All the St. John's Wort in the world will not help you when you are pouring several cups of coffee down your system. Caffeine also puts unnecessary stress on the kidneys. Check with your local health food store for every coffee substitute available and buy a sample of each one. Take them home and try them all. Taking coffee, artificial sweeteners, nondairy creamers, or even low-fat milk out of your diet will improve your health immeasurably. Be aware that you are withdrawing from an addictive substance when you stop drinking coffee (I call coffee the largest legal drug in America.) Someone who has consumed four to eight cups of coffee daily can expect to experience headaches, cold or sinus infection symptoms, constipation, drowsiness or nervous jitters as a result of cold-turkey caffeine withdrawal. These indicate that your body is attempting to cleanse itself of the poisonous effects of years of caffeine intake. Try to remember the zest and energy that you had as a child, and be reassured that they are still available, once the false high of caffeine is withdrawn and the body cleansed.

If you are addicted to coffee, I suggest that initially you cut back rather than going cold turkey. For example, if you normally consume eight cups a day, cut back to three. Each cup should be half filled with coffee and half with Jason Winters Tea. After about one week, decrease the amount of coffee by half again, and eliminate the coffee entirely within another week. (Decaffeinated coffee still contains some caffeine—in fact, anything that doesn't say "caffeine free" should be avoided.) I drink four to eight cups of Jason Winters Tea each day.

If you rely on coffee to stimulate your colon each morning, as many people do, an herbal laxative may be advisable for the first few days of withdrawal. Adding more raw fruit to your diet will also help.

The tea's herbs were originally combined by Jason Winters, who was the stunt man for movie star Audie Murphy. His fascinating book, *The Jason Winters Story,*[2] relates his experience with cancer and how that experience led him to this wonderful herbal combination. Jason had a small bump on the side of his throat that he ignored for a long period of time. As the lump grew larger, his friends finally insisted that he have it looked at by a medical doctor. During a "minor" biopsy, they discovered that Jason had cancer of the larynx, the pharynx, the jaw, the tongue and the area surrounding his heart. After six hours of surgery, they sewed him back up and gave him three months to live.

After recovering from surgery, he grew increasingly interested in the healing power of herbs, and traveled around the world looking for a class of herbs called blood cleansers. When he arrived in China, where he found the third and last ingredient, his health had deteriorated to the point that he was in a wheelchair. He returned home and immediately began taking the three blood cleansers— initially, brewing, and drinking the herbs separately. But one day he was lying on the kitchen floor too weak to get up and wash the pot, so he simply threw in all three ingredients and brewed them together. With the first sip, he could tell it was different. He drank a gallon that day and a gallon each day for three months thereafter—six months later, he was diagnosed as being cancer free.

Along with this marvelous tea, he used other herbs to clean the accumulation of mucous that coated the walls of his colon from years of eating meat, milk, and white bread. And he fired every doctor that had told him he was going to die. The combination of the blood-cleansing tea, other herbs, and positive thinking (Jason is a big advocate of positive thinking.) brought him back to perfect health. To this day he travels the world lecturing on the power of herbs to restore health.

The Holistic View of B-Complex, Stress, and Bursitis

If patients walk into my office complaining of too much stress, or if they tell me that their nerves are fried, they can't keep up with their jobs, run the household, or pay the bills, I will advise them that B-complex is the perfect nutrition. These vitamins won't reduce their stress, but they will help them stay calm and handle the load in a more relaxed manner.

I had not seen Carolyn for over a year. She originally came in with low-back pain, and I gave her a massage-like naprapathic treatment, some calcium minerals and told her to take a couple of Masada baths. It seemed to help, and she didn't need to see me again for eight months. When she finally returned, she sounded a little raspy. She had a recurring bout with bronchitis, and though she had just gotten off of a series of antibiotics, she was thinking about going back to her medical doctor for another prescription. Of course, her real reason for coming to me was muscular-skeletal. She had pain in the left shoulder where the bursa is located. The bursa is a sac that surrounds the joint, and inflammation of this sack is called *bursitis* (In fact, "*-itis*" means inflammation of a body part). At any rate, lifting and carrying her two-and-half-year-old son may have caused, and certainly hadn't helped, her condition, which she'd had for a month.

Human energy begins at the core of our being. For men this is the heart. For women it is the female organs which then push this vital energy to the heart. From the heart it flows out in all directions. I began Carolyn's treatment with soft tissue massage on the center of her back at the level of her heart. Even if a patient's problem is in the shoulder, elbow, or fingers, I always start at this core and work out. While I massaged the tight stiff muscles that lay along Carolyn's spine, we talked about bronchitis (inflammation of the bronchial tubes).

Because my first objective is always to stop whatever is assaulting the body, I suggested that during periods of congestion and additional mucus in the body, she avoid foods that promote this condition. Dairy, beef, white bread products, peanut butter, and ice cold drinks must not be eaten when the lungs, sinuses, and glands are congested. She said she puts just a little cream or milk in her morning coffee, "not enough to bother anyone." I reminded her that the body's reaction to this everyday assault of dairy must be considered similar to an allergic reaction. For example, if she were allergic to bees instead of dairy, it wouldn't matter if it were a big bee or an itty bitty bee. That itty bitty bee that flies into her coffee each morning before stinging her is still an assault on her overworked system. Whether it is dairy or a bee sting, the body jump-starts the immune system into full throttle when attacked. And when that attack continues day after day, even though at a low level, the body can be irritated enough to cause adrenal exhaustion.

The adrenals, a pair of glands that sit on top of the kidneys, are the military control system that ward off assaults to the body. They get our muscles pumped with blood and ready to flee as soon as we see a bear in the woods. They also shut down available blood to our digestive systems, or any other system that can't help us run as fast as we can to escape the sharp claws of Mr. Bear. Even when the assault is less traumatic (*e.g.*, an allergy to dairy or white bread products), the adrenal glands still prepare for battle, this time against the offensive substance. The stress of these continuous attacks (for months or even years) leads to perpetual battle-alarm responses and a very tired adrenal system. I suggested that instead of dairy,

Carolyn should substitute rice or soy milk in her coffee (I person-ally prefer the flavor of rice milk.)

Carolyn, having been to Weight Watchers, found that she had trouble staying away from chocolate, and asked if chocolate could also cause a mucus reaction. Again I said yes, explaining the yin and yang of food. Very hard, solid, dense foods such as salt, beef, pork, chicken, fish, dairy, nuts, beans, seeds, and grains are clas-sified as having a yang quality. Foods considered to be more yin have qualities of lightness, airiness, and fluffiness. Foods possessing these qualities in a descending order are drugs (both recreational and prescription), nonfood foods such as chemicals and preser-vatives and then alcohol, coffee, carbonated drinks, sugar, candy, fruit juice, and fruit. Then there are vegetables in a descending order, from those with a light, airy quality such as leafy greens to those with a more hard, condensed quality such as carrots.

The body always balances the yin with the yang [**See Yin and Yang food chart page 97.**] If you eat a meal of pork or steak, it is perfectly natural to want an accompanying glass of wine, cold beer, carbon-ated drink, ice water, or a dessert with sugar. The heavy yang meats balance nicely with the expansive alcohol, coffee, carbonated bever-ages, or sugar. Most vegetarians (*i.e.,* those who eat grains, nuts, and seeds) never feel compelled to drink alcohol because their balance is so much lower on the yin/yang scale. They find that fruit is as expansive as they need to balance out the yang choices of grain, nuts, and seeds.

Carolyn and I determined that she might be drawn toward choco-late because she ate a lot of dense animal foods from the yang side of the chart. Eating salt, steak, lamb, and/or pork led her to want something more yin to balance it out. Chocolate would sustain that balance. Maintaining this balance is done without conscious thought on Carolyn's (or anyone else's) part. Every time I have a piece of lamb, it's nice to have a glass of wine with it. But, chil-dren can't have wine to balance out steak, pork, or chicken, so they are drawn—almost compelled—toward sugary desserts and too

YIN AND YANG FOOD CHART

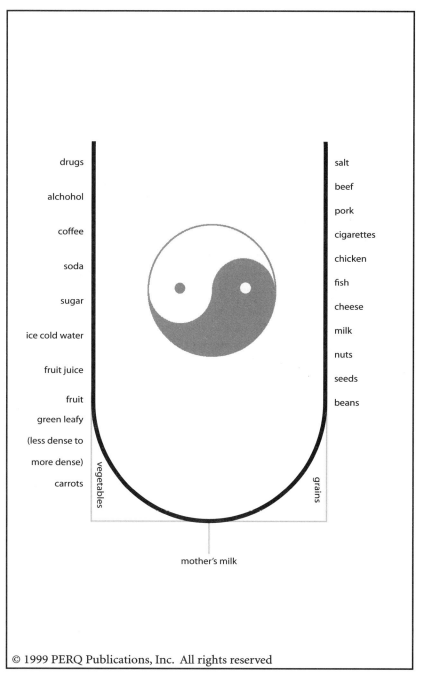

much chocolate. If they are continually fed a yang diet of heavy meat, eventually they will be drawn, as teenagers, to drugs or alcohol to balance out this heavy meat intake.

I also pointed out to Carolyn that the sugar in chocolate strips her body's B-complex vitamins—her stress protectors. Sugar irritates the myelin sheath that surrounds each nerve, causing inflammation and altering the messages that flow along nerve roots. These altered transmissions translate into nervousness in any stressful situation.

As we talked more about stress and its effect on the body, Carolyn told me that her mother had died in September and described her mother's degeneration from cirrhosis of the liver. Carolyn had not really been aware that her mother was dying. Although she had been diagnosed with the disease 15 years earlier, she seemed to have recovered. But suddenly, her whole abdominal area became bloated because her liver could no longer move fluids properly. Once in the hospital, her decline was very rapid. Within three days, Carolyn's mother was dead.

With this last piece of information, the little medical light went on in my head. "Of course, of course!" I said, "The lungs hold sadness!" Carolyn had contracted bronchitis in January and was still suffering from it at the end of June when she arrived in my office. She was not able to come to terms with the family's decision to decline any extraordinary steps to keep her mom alive, and she felt terribly responsible. Carolyn was torn apart emotionally about the rapid decisions she had to make, and she was incredibly upset and saddened by the very sudden death. Her mother was only 64, so she died long before anyone would think it was her time to go. In addition, she was on so many drugs that she was unable to speak. Able only to write notes to her children, she left so much unsaid— so many emotions to choke Carolyn's sad lungs.

I then understood that Carolyn's stubborn lung congestion was really her sadness refusing to let go. She needed to read *You Can't Afford the Luxury of a Negative Thought,* by John Roberts.[3] This book teaches how to stop the never-ending series of messages in our heads telling ourselves that we have made the wrong decisions—"I could have done this," or "I could have done that." Roberts instructs the reader to say, "Stop!" right out loud to this negative internal dialogue.

Carolyn needed to stop reliving the agony over and over, so I encouraged her to imagine the favorite places her mother liked to go. For Carolyn's mom, it was a trip the whole family took to a gambling boat in Illinois. I told her to imagine her mother standing by the boat's railing, smiling and waving. I suggested that Carolyn picture herself putting dollars in her mother's hand because she was a happy winner. Carolyn needed to tell herself "stop" every time she started to play the death scenario in her head, and to imagine that her mom was now peaceful and okay.

Carolyn thought that her mother probably would be unhappy with all her negative fussing. She imagined that her mother would probably yell at her. But no, I insisted, "Your mother is the one who pushed you through the door of my office to get help." I pointed out that maybe this whole drama occurred so that Carolyn would stop dwelling in the negative, churning up despair again and again, and creating poison in her body. Without the pain that Carolyn had created for herself, she would never have yearned for a new way of looking at life. So pain becomes a gift. It is only when our despair becomes painful enough that we take that first step toward help.

Carolyn told me that she felt an incredible calm enter the room just before her mother was about to take her last breath. I told her that as her mother was passing away, her spirit came and hugged her, gave her warmth, and whispered in her ear that she was going to be fine. She was going to a better place, and Carolyn just had to trust those things. She had to trust that her path would lead her to a new way of thinking—a new way of letting go. If her mother's death was to be the push that she required, then she needed to thank her mom. She needed to rely on her inner voice and go with the flow.

Carolyn left my office teary-eyed, but feeling much better. Although her lungs were still congested, her shoulder felt good. In hand, she had a laundry list of health-food-store items, including Echinacea, a natural herbal antibiotic for her lung congestion, and rice milk as an alternative to mucus-forming dairy products. Her second stop was the library to pick up *You Can't Afford the Luxury of a Negative Thought*. She was to check back with me to see how the shoulder was doing. I wished her luck with her new way of being.

Nerves, Depression, and the Right Herbs

Which organ do you think holds depression? Can we cut into the body, take out the offender, and lighten the load to free ourselves from the weight of depression? And, of course, it is a great weight. It keeps women in bed, unable to accomplish the normal tasks of daily living. It even prevents women from making simple decisions. So, shall we look in the brain? Should we look in the heart? No. We need to look at the very center of each and every woman. We need to look in the female organs.

An important oriental principle says that the uterus is considered the primary center or core of a woman's being. When female reproductive organs are weak, when a woman does not receive proper nutrition, or when nurturing love does not surround her, her entire female system weakens. When female organs are bombarded with artificial sprays and scents, harmful cleansing products, and/or toxic sanitary tampons, then the system grows weaker each year. If the job a woman holds does not support the premise that she is an important nurturing component in the lives of everyone around her, her uterus will grow weaker still.

The energy from the female reproductive organs is directly linked to, or feeds, the heart's energy. If the heart becomes weak, it is a direct result of a decrease in energy from the uterus. Chinese medical theory views weakness of the heart, as a result of female organ deficiency, as the primary cause of depression. The Chinese use a two-thousand-year-old formula, called Women's Precious, to balance that deficiency. It contains the herbs angelica pubescens, panax ginseng, angelica sinenses, dong quai, and saliva militiorrhiza.

According to Daniel Reed's book, *Chinese Herbal Medicine*, angelica pubescens is a pungent and bitter herb used to drive out "wind-damp" excess. It regulates and moves energy and stagnated blood, while relieving pain and stiffness in the lower back and knees. Its effects are described as anti-rheumatic and analgesic.[4]

Angelica sinenses is a sweet and pungent, yet warming, herb. It is considered to be both the ultimate female tonic and also an excellent blood tonic, beneficial to men as well as women. It is said to warm up the inner organs, improve circulation, beautify the skin, and hasten the healing of cuts and wounds. In cases of anemia, the herb has blood-building qualities when cooked. Also called Tang Kuei, angelica sinenses is additionally an emennagogue and is used to promote circulation, especially for menstrual disorders or blood deficiencies. It has analgesic, sedative, and laxative qualities.[5] And Reed also reports that the herb can be used for painful scarring from traumatic injuries and for post-natal abdominal pain.[6]

Saliva militiorrhiza is a bitter, slightly cold root which has an affinity for the heart. It promotes circulation and dissolves blood clots. It not only tones the blood, but is also described by Reed as a blood refrigerant. Its indications include amenorrhoea (an absence or lack of menstrual flow), metrorrhoea (bleeding from the uterus, other than the normal menstrual flow), and post-natal abdominal pains. Other indications include poor circulation, abdominal and chest pains, blood clots, heart palpitations, and insomnia. Also called dan shen, it is commonly used to reduce inflammation of the liver and is excellent for coronary diseases.[7]

Panax ginseng grows wild in the mountains of the northeastern provinces of China. Its root, used to tone the primordial energy of the body, is also utilized as a tonic specifically for the lungs and spleen and to nourish vital fluids. In addition, it is (you may or may not be happy to hear) an aphrodisiac. Ginseng regulates blood pressure and blood sugar. It promotes secretion of sexual hormones in men and women, and promotes the production of blood by toning vital qui energy. "Strictly avoid tea (black) and turnips when using ginseng."[8]

This sacred herb (which can be taken in the Women's Precious formula or occasionally taken alone) will increase the strength of the heart. It is characterized as a harmonizing tonic, helping to improve coronary circulation and normalizing arterial pressure. Because ginseng helps the body produce more red blood cells, oxygen, which is carried by these cells, is also greatly increased. I advise my patients that getting more blood to the site of an injury also means more oxygen, and that translates into less pain when suffering from muscular-skeletal injuries.

Ginseng is also a stress adapter, or more technically, an adaptogen—a term given to any substance that can increase the body's general resistance (*i.e.,* make it work more efficiently and fend off disease better). Ginseng's root, which is often, remarkably, shaped like a man, has been called a gift from the gods, bestowed on men and woman to give them strength. When I was pregnant, I used it to fortify both my baby and me—it was the only herb my Chinese healer allowed me to take during that time.

Ginseng is a blood-cleansing herb that will pull toxins out of cellular spaces and fat cells. Because of this property, a large initial dose will cause a tremendous headache as the toxins enter the blood stream. If I start patients off with a separate ginseng extract, the first day they are to take one-fifth the normal dose. The next day, the dose is increased in the morning and afternoon. Gradually, they work their way up to between 30 and 60 drops daily, depending on their condition.

Always drink ginseng warm, or take Women's Precious formula with warm water. The formula is available in compressed pellets that are usually swallowed whole, first thing in the morning (taken with the warm water, of course).

The herb has healing benefits when warm, but can stress the vital energy of the kidneys when cold. Ginseng Rush is a bubbly, cold soda-pop-like drink that can be purchased from the health food store. It tastes great, but ice cold, it doesn't have the blood-cleansing or strengthening properties of warm ginseng. Besides, the cold will irritate nerve tissue. However, anyone with mucus accumulations in the lungs (asthma, bronchitis, or chest colds) should avoid ginseng altogether.

If I'm driving and the warning light comes on telling me that my car is almost out of gas, it's not a good idea for me to put on rose colored glasses so I can't see the warning light. That's what Prozac is—a pair of rose colored glasses. It is a drug that binds receptors so that we cannot feel depression. The body is incredibly wise, and we should always honor and trust its wisdom before taking anyone's advise about cutting off its signals. Rather, we should learn from these signals that we are not in our steady, or homeostatic, state of optimal health. We should provide the right balance, whether it's nutrients (B-complex), Chinese herbs (Women's Precious herbal formula), counseling, or hypnosis. We need to take a good look at what our bodies need. Pain, discomfort, and depression are all signals that we are avoiding something that needs to be addressed. Change is the result of discomfort felt a little too long.

Chamomile: An Herb for Depression and the Nerves

The herb chamomile, is classified as a nervine, which means it contains all the right combination of vitamins and minerals for nutrition to address any problem that involves the nerves. Chamomile is simply the Great Spirit's good food for someone in the depressed state. Make one strong cup right before bed if you have trouble sleeping—a condition associated with depression. In fact, if you awake in the middle of the night because your mind is churning, worrying, and replaying your daily problems, another cup of very strong chamomile tea will help put you right back to sleep.

Chamomile is also a carminative; it aids in digestion and also has some mild antibiotic properties. I suggest one half cup of chamomile tea before a meal, and one half to one cup twenty minutes after a meal to help digest and assimilate all the nutrients you've eaten.

When dealing with depression, perspective is also very important. I have made the most effective changes—taken my best spiritual steps forward—at the end of a depressed state, like an alcoholic who needs to hit bottom in order to take the first step up the recovery ladder. I advise my patients to stand up and move to a different chair in the room when they are examining a difficult emotional situation. Because every life experience is a blessing, we must get a different perspective. We must understand that a change in a job or living arrangements can be seen as a positive—seen as the spirit moving us to a new phase in our lives. If we examine every depressing situation in order to find the positive, we will not be knocked down so low each time depression knocks at our door. The more we practice this, the more attention we will pay; therefore, we'll be able to recognize needed change before we get to that terribly depressed state.

Nerves, Tingling Hands, Carpal-Tunnel, and Thoracic Outlet Syndromes

The body is wise. Every health issue is an example of our intimate communication with this beautiful shell we walk around in. Our job is to learn the language, but it takes a lifetime.

Consider the body's wisdom as it relates to the heart, depression, and carpal tunnel. Although a woman's female organs are the primary center, the heart plays an important role. Because the heart keeps us working every day, it uses tremendous amounts of energy and strength to pump nutrients to every part of our bodies, from our hair follicles to our toenails. Eating too much red meat, standing for long hours under fluorescent lights, or being a workaholic puts tremendous stress on the heart. And most of the time it responds without the slightest moan or groan. Then we add the standard American diet of three to four cups of coffee a day (which strips the nerve's ability to transmit signals properly), and food that arrives at the grocery lacking 50 percent of its vitamin content. This abuse can occasionally cause us to experience numb and tingling hands while we sleep. Ignore the problem, and the body will shout a little louder by making our hands numb during waking hours.

My patients complain that most numbness begins while they are engaged in their favorite activities. One of my friends who plays polo says his right hand goes numb when he tries to grasp his mallet tightly. Another patient who crochets tells me that as soon as she starts working on her favorite flower pattern, the first two fingers of her right hand start to tingle. The doctor will say that it's carpal tunnel. This is a condition in which the ligaments that form a small tunnel-like structure in the wrist, allowing blood vessels and nerves to go the palm and fingers of the hand, have tightened up. The doctor gives the patient a wrist brace and the insurance company a bill. Meanwhile, the patient waits.

When the hand and fingers go numb, it's because the heart is not up to full strength, so the body makes a decision to conserve the heart's vital energy and lets the extremities do without. I'm sure your dad, grandfather, or uncle has said to you when you've bumped or cut a leg or finger, "Not to worry. It's a long way from the heart." Oh, the wisdom of these cute little sayings.

When you grab that glass of wine, cup of coffee, and/or piece of white-flour bread or bagel, your fingers tend to get numb or tingly. While asleep, you lie on your shoulders or on your side, compressing the nerves and blood vessels that travel through your shoulders. Upon waking, your hands are asleep, and you can't seem to get any feeling back. When you cut the circulation off in the front of the shoulders and your hands tingle, this is sometimes diagnosed as thoracic outlet syndrome. Whether it is carpal tunnel or thoracic outlet syndrome, the first thing you must do is move toward a more vegetarian diet. Fish is fine, a little chicken is okay, but beef, pork, and lamb are definitely out when you're trying to reenergize the heart so that it has the strength to pump blood out to the tips of the fingers. In this instance, red meat is definitely not in the diet plan.

B-complex is nutrition for nerves. If you're going to use a supplement, my first choice for perfect well-rounded nerve nutrition is Complete B-Complex by Rainbow Light. The adult dosage suggested on the bottle is three capsules in the morning. Because B-complex is an energizing vitamin, it's best to take it in the morning. Some patients have said that it keeps them awake if taken in the evening, and it has the same effect on me. So, as a rule of thumb, take minerals before going to sleep at night and vitamins in the morning.

A tight muscle spasm can restrict blood flow or nerve transmissions to the hands. Calcium minerals help to keep muscles calm; therefore, it is an important component in keeping shoulder and arm muscles relaxed. The recommended daily allowance (RDA) for calcium, set by the Food and Drug Administration, is 800 milligrams a day. But, for an adult with carpal tunnel, I routinely raise that dose to between 1,200 and 1,500 milligrams. Research has found that the combination of calcium and magnesium prevents kidney stones, so most calcium supplements include magnesium. In the case of dark-green herbal supplements (such as Cal-Mineral, which I use in my practice), the Great Spirit conveniently supplies the magnesium. If, by chance, you have kidney stones, seek the advice of a medical doctor who has some knowledge of nutrition and herbs.

Good Old-Fashioned Rubdowns and Exercises

Any insufficiency of the heart manifested as carpal tunnel, thoracic outlet syndrome, or numb and tingling hands needs a trained naprapath, naprapathic-chiropractor, massage therapist, or a massage-oriented chiropractor to massage the muscles in the back that lie at the level of the heart, to massage the shoulders and arms all the way down to the hands, and to rotate the arms in large circles to promote good circulation. The goal is to release the tension that surrounds the heart and restricts blood flow to the hands,

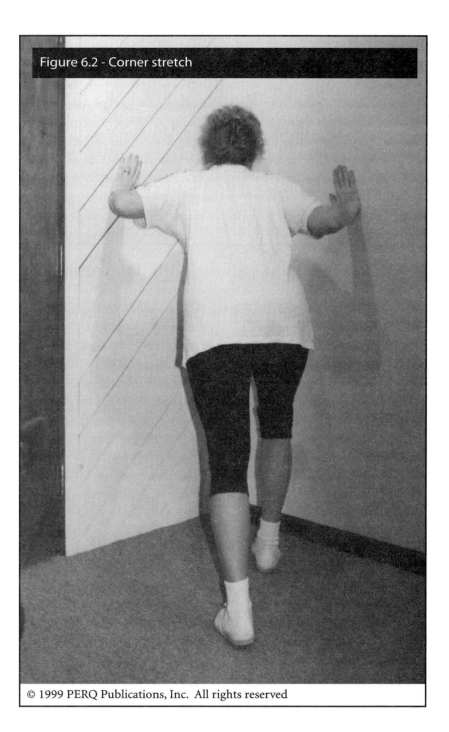

Figure 6.2 - Corner stretch

which have acupuncture points and reflex points that correspond to other areas of the body. Massaging the entire hand and the wrist helps to pull circulation down into the fingers.

Exercises that pull the shoulders apart and backward are also helpful in releasing tension surrounding the heart. One such exercise is the corner stretch, which can be done two or three times a day. [**Figure 6.2**] Go to a corner and place both hands on the walls at the height of your shoulders. Place your legs in a lunge position, which means that one leg is directly under the center of your body and the other is a foot and a half behind your body. Lunge forward until your face and chest are a few inches from the corner, making sure your elbows are pointing out on each side like bird wings. This pose stretches the large muscles in the front of the chest called the pectorals, major and minor. Slowly ease into the position as far as you can comfortably stretch, breathe deeply, and after approximately one minute, stretch a little farther into the position. Hold the stretch for approximately two minutes. Then slowly stand upright, switch legs, and repeat the entire procedure. To avoid straining muscle tissues, it is important not to bounce in and out of position, but to move slowly and gradually, and to breathe slowly and deeply.

Another helpful exercise for pulling the shoulders apart and backwards is to interlace your fingers behind your body at the waist and raise the interlaced fingers as high as you can with your arms straight and elbows locked. Yes, *behind* your back. [**Figure 6.3**] Hold this position for approximately one to three minutes. This procedure can cause numbness and tingling in your fingers. When that occurs, hold the position for another ten seconds, then shake out your hands and try again. If you repeat this exercise twice a day, within two weeks circulation will improve, the numbness and tingling may disappear, and the length of time you can hold your arms up will increase. Each time you do this exercise, you are stretching and opening the circulation route through the shoulders and increasing the potential for vital circulation.

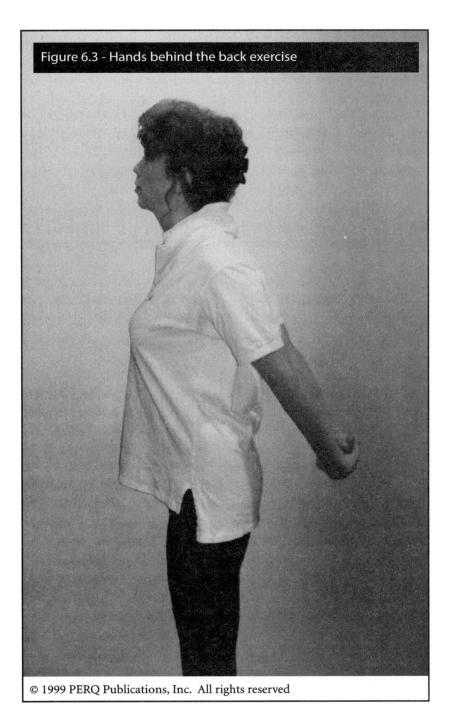

Figure 6.3 - Hands behind the back exercise

Body language is very important with carpal tunnel. When the shoulders slump forward and the head bends down, our body is saying, "I'm trying to protect my heart." The premise is that the heart is weakened, so it is not pumping blood to the fingers. Whether it's job stress, emotional stress because of a personal relationship, or any other problem, we slope our shoulders forward to cut off circulation to the extremities, and in that way protect the heart. Being aware of our posture, focusing on pulling those shoulders back, and doing the exercises are the first steps toward better health. Trying some of the following affirmations also helps: "I am now going to take better care of my heart." "I am now going to eat better for my heart." "I am now going to look positively at all the emotional issues that surround me in order to have a more open loving heart." "My hands won't get tingly. I'll be able to touch and hold and grab all the possibilities the world has to offer."

1. Louise Hay, *Heal Your Body* (Carson, California: Hay House, Inc., 1988), p. 99.

2. Jason Wingers, *The Jason Winters Story.*

3. John Roberts, *You Can't Afford the Luxury of a Negative Thought.*

4. Daniel Reed, *Chinese Herbal Medicine* (Boston: Shambala Publications, Inc., 1994), p. 112.

5. Ron Teeguarden with Caroline Davies, *Chinese Tonic Herbs* (Japan Publications, Inc., 1984), pp. 85-86.

6. Reed, p. 151.

7. Reed, p. 129.

8. Reed, p. 144.

Chapter 7

Recharging Your Batteries

Run down batteries

Everyone experiences this condition at the end of a long day or after a particularly stressful event. A day off usually brings us back to full steam. But what if *your* full steam still means that you're tired by five o'clock every evening, or you're tired when you awaken after a full eight hours sleep? Why do some people always seem to have vibrant energy and others look and feel a little old for their age? "It's in the genes," you say. "My dad had gray hair by the time he was 38. I'm sure that I'll look mature by that age, too. You can't fight genetics, you know."

But, I know *you*. You're the one who absolutely cannot get up without that cup of coffee each morning. You start the day in slow gear or, maybe, no gear at all. Remember the spark of life you had as a kid without that cup of mocha or espresso? That energy— *natural*, not caffeine-generated—is yours for the asking. Do you want it badly enough? Or are you comfortable in your present routine?

The principle of inertia says that an object (or a middle-aged human being) tends to continue along the same path unless acted upon by an outside force. In other words, it's easier for us to keep doing the same old things than it is to initiate movement in a new direction. Most of us need to get sick in order to make major life changes—our health becomes very precious when it begins to dwindle. Even then, the average person only has the stamina to maintain a new diet plan for about three days before resuming some of the old habits. But the mere fact that you considered a change is wonderful, for you are on the brink of becoming more of the person you want to be. A little time passes and again, you strive to make another attempt at self-change. This time one piece of it sticks. Before long, you realize that you're eating less beef and pork—those heavy animal proteins. Someone hands you a cup of coffee and you decline because you've already had your limit of one cup a day. You would really prefer tea and of course, you've brought your own Jason Winters's tea bag along with you.

Having been at this point myself, I thought you would like to know some of the things I've discovered to increase my energy potential. Too many of my patients buy a general multiple vitamin at the local grocery store, take it for a couple of months, and are never really sure if it has any affect on them. That is a waste of vital self-change energy. So, I'm going to tell you about those things that will make you feel good right away—that will make you say, "Wow!" because you actually *feel the effects*.

The Breath

Let's start with your very essence—your breath. If you begin your day with a cleansing breath, you enable your lungs to cast off stagnated air that has accumulated overnight.

Begin by inhaling and exhaling deeply through your nose for three complete breaths. On the fourth breath, inhale very deeply and hold it for about a second. Then exhale through your mouth, which is pursed in the shape of a small "o." Exhale forcibly in three separate bursts of air. There are three lobes or separate compartments to each lung. Imagine that each part of your forced exhalation is cleaning out all the stagnant air trapped in the farthest reaches of each of these lobes. This cleansing-breath exercise can be done when you get up, before you go to bed, or as often as you like during the day.

When you feel tired, you can gather energy with the cleansing-breath exercise I just described. Then inhale deeply, hold your breath for about three seconds, or three heartbeats. Exhale fully through your nose. Repeat this process a couple of times and then do a body check. Mentally scan tension, tiredness and available attitude energy. Did the heavy tired feeling leave your chest? Do you feel like continuing with whatever project you've planned? If not, repeat both the cleansing-breath and the energizing-breath exercises.

Affirmations

It is my job to help you restore that zest for life. Of course, you must make the initial effort toward greater health and vitality. Most of the folks that walk through my door are already sick. I've heard it said that disease begins first with a thought such as, "I'm working too many hours for the salary I was quoted." If the thought is uncomfortable, erroneous, restricted, or does not fit in with the universal truth, it will lead to stress, depression, anxiety, or anger. If these emotions are not addressed, but are instead left to fester, physical illness will eventually ensue. Carrying the weight of the world on overworked shoulders will cause you to wake up with a shoulder that you can't move or lower back pain that won't allow you to take another step toward that debilitating job situation.

"But what about the time I stubbed my toe on the couch and fractured it in two places? That can't be due to negative emotions, too, could it?" I refer to those kinds of situations as just a little of life's acupuncture, with a very large needle—the couch—trying to stimulate a very stuck energy flow! Positive thinking, especially positive affirmations, repeated again and again, can elevate any mood, can change disappointment, anger, jealousy, or sorrow into a more positive state of mind. When the negative voice inside your head says repeatedly that the man you're living with is treating you awfully, that you should be making more money, that your boss has not seen your full potential, the whole room fills with vibrating atoms of negativity, bringing you further and further down. Repeating affirmations can change the whole situation: can take the downward spiral of your job and send it soaring up toward the heavens with new possibilities, new raises, new outlooks on careers. It can open up the possibilities for transformation. One negative thought is like the locomotive of a train pulling one railroad car of negativity after another, until the entire room is so filled with negativity that those of us who can feel, touch and see it, can hardly enter the room.

Today must be the day that you start shutting off the negative voice in your head. However, developing the habit is not always easy. Because the subconscious wants to keep us in a pattern that we've already established, positive affirmations can be easily forgotten. Write affirmative notes to yourself that are applicable to your present situation. Post them on the rearview mirror of your car (a wonderful place to put a positive note or a protection prayer), on the mirror in the bathroom, or above the coat hooks in the closet—anywhere they can be seen on a daily basis. Stop a minute, take a deep breath, relax, and say your positive prayer—it's a wonderful habit to get into. It will open up your life to so many new possibilities. Rather than continuing to live with the negativity that keeps you afraid to try new directions, you will begin to create the life that you've always wanted.

Liquids

My grandfather started his day off with two cups of hot water to get his intestines going every morning. Tap water was okay then, but today bottled water is a better choice. If you insist on some flavor, try Jason Winters Tea. This is the one product I recommend that 99 percent of my patients try and use consistently. Its rich roasted flavor provides a wonderful replacement for coffee. Both men and women seem to enjoy the taste and the caffeine-free energy.

Jason Winters Tea contains red clover, Indian sage, and a special spice from China. These blood-cleansing ingredients attach to the cellular waste products and toxic elements floating around in the blood and pull them from your system. This affords the rest of your cells the opportunity to accomplish many other tasks than continually picking up your body's garbage. More cells are available to help you think, move, digest, and carry out other bodily functions more rapidly. The end results are more available energy and a longer, healthier life.

Try Jason Winters in the tea bags first to see if the taste agrees with you. The tea bags contain a preroasted blend, whereas the loose-leaf tea packaged in the large containers has a milder, more leafy-herbal taste. Fill a quart pot with four cups of water, and boil for about five minutes. Dr. Deepak Chopra believes, based on ancient ayurvedic holistic healing practices, that the energy required to boil water still resides in the water as long as it retains its heat.[1] While the water is still boiling, pour it into a thermos with two bags of Jason Winters Tea, and take the thermos along with you for the day.

Some of you don't want to give up the taste of coffee each morning. Your elbows may ache, your hands may go numb each night, or sciatic nerve pain may plague you as you drive to work, but you still don't want to give up that steaming hot cup of coffee. For you, I have a compromise. Pour one-half to three-quarters cup of coffee and top it off with Jason Winters Tea. You will get the taste you're addicted to and the tea will help clean up some of the damage the coffee is creating. Two weeks down the road, reduce the ratio of coffee to tea. As you wean yourself from the caffeine, you may get headaches, stuffy sinuses, or a full-blown cold. You are withdrawing from an addictive substance, which is never an easy thing to do. However, it's much easier to withdraw from one-third cup of coffee than from three or four full cups. Whether you drink the tea plain or add coffee to it, you will love its energy potential and flavor. Good luck!

Vitamins and Minerals

"Vitamins in the morning and minerals at bedtime"—that's the rule in my practice. The vitamin to choose first thing in the morning is B-complex (the B vitamins combat stress and provide proper nutrition for any nerve-related problem.) However, because they are high-potential-energy vitamins, I advise my patients not to take them at bedtime if they have trouble sleeping.

My favorite is Complete B-Complex, formulated by the Rainbow Light Company. Its food-based supplement has no caffeine, but contains bee pollen, spirulina (micro-algae), barley grass, and wheat germ—the "superfoods" I often recommend as regular additions to the diet. Ginseng, dong quai root, ginger root, orange root, hawthorn, and schisandra fruit make up the herbal blend of the formula. B-Complex also contains vitamins C, B-1, B-2, B-3, B-5, B-6, B-12, beta-carotene, folic acid, and biotin. Its mineral content includes calcium and magnesium, zinc, iron, and potassium with choline. It contains lecithin, a great emulsifier, which combats heart disease by keeping the arteries slippery clean. And it contains bioflavonoids, which cool inflammation. But guess what? Rainbow Light's B-Complex is expensive, of course. If your health food store does not carry this brand, ask them to order it. It's worth the extra money to have a product that consistently relieves the harmful effects of stress, restores vitality, and works well with radiating sciatic nerve problems and hand and foot numbness.

When you start to clean up your body, sugar is one of the first items that must go. You can add all the vitamins you want, but to see vibrant, healthy results more quickly, you must also delete the harmful things. Sugar-ladened fruit punches, fruit juices with added corn sweeteners, and artificially sweetened fruit drinks do not meet my "if-the-Great-Spirit-made-it-it's-okay-to-eat-or-drink" criterion.

I've found some pretty tasty substitutes for those over-sweetened drinks. Recharge, for example is a great tasting noncarbonated beverage that also replaces electrolytes. Not only is it a great juice for kids or adults any time of day, it is also perfect for drinking after athletic workouts. Electrolytes are the minerals that make our bodily systems operate efficiently. They are also the same minerals that we need and get in dark-green leafy foods. Recharge replaces these minerals lost when we exercise.

We need minerals to move our muscles as we lift and walk all day, and to help our muscles *not* move. People who are slaves to their computers and telephones are in constant need of additional minerals to replace those lost from the hard work of maintaining one position for hours. With the strenuous demands my job places on my muscles, I can easily go through one to two quarts of this marvelous drink daily. Children who are building bones and muscles and developing all their organ systems can easily drink a couple of quarts daily. This healthy product, which comes in lemon-lime, orange, and tropical flavors can probably only be found at your local health food store.

Power Foods—the Great Spirit's Mysterious Spark

"Power foods" are what I call certain foods that not only provide vitamins and minerals, but also deliver that mysterious spark— that elusive quality—that is life itself. In a laboratory, scientists can add all the right elements to create sea water, but marine life cannot survive in it unless a touch of real sea water is added. That same principle can be applied to our food choices. Whole and unprocessed foods provide us with more robust energy and that extra spark of vitality that some people seem to beam with and others wish they had. Because that vibrant spark comes from Mother Nature, let's go back to the garden, where we can create our full energy potential.

Many ancient healers, medicine men of the Native American, tribes, and curandaros and shamans of South America respect plant life and its ability to heal. Although it sounds simple, we should not take the word *respect* too lightly. Many of these healers view plants as vibrant, sentient beings, capable of emotional reactions and possessing a spirit that sustains life. To them, human life embodies that spirit and is positively enhanced by it when we eat plants. Therefore, respect for that life form involves asking its permission to utilize its energy potential and thanking it afterwards for the sacrifice it's made.

As children, most of us were taught to thank God, or the Great Spirit, for providing the food we were about to eat. Children and adults repeat their thanks without grasping the tremendous, yet simple, concept that the spark of the Great Spirit's energy these plants have to offer is precisely what they are searching for when they buy that new multiple vitamin supplement, that colloidal mineral drink, or that power shake. Why the search? Because they are eating dead food—and *dead* is precisely its condition. The combined amount of electrical energy used to process, grind, mix, spit out, and mold those sugar-ladened breakfast cereals has canceled out all the energy potential the food had to offer. That vital energy no longer follows a plant to the supermarket, into our homes, our salad bowls, and down into our stomachs.

"But how can I be in California encouraging that vital spirit that occupies each cabbage, turnip, and green bean to accompany me home?" you ask. "I have enough trouble remembering to eat well, let alone having to worry about not insulting each plant I eat simply because I've never asked its permission to pick it. Now you have gone too far!" Okay, it's a philosophical notion that perhaps has limited application, but any food that *you* can raise *yourself* puts you one step ahead of multilevel vitamin salespeople with their inflated prices.

Try sticking Swiss chard seeds in a window box or patio planter to grow your own delicious greens if a full blown garden is beyond your time and energy. Before picking a few leaves to steam for dinner, declare your faith in the power that plants have to feed and heal us, and thank the plant's spirit. Before picking any vegetable from my garden or wild edible herbal weed growing in the forest, I say the following prayer: "Great Spirit, I am the one that walks the fields to gather the medicine to heal the sickness of the people.

I thank the spirit of this plant, and I have faith with all my heart that it will both feed and heal the sickness of the people. Thank you, Great Spirit." This prayer was taught to me by the marvelous healer, Dr. Rosita Arvigo, a naprapath and one of the world's leading experts in medicinal herbs from the rain forests of South America. Dr. Arvigo learned this ancient Mayan ritual of saying prayers when gathering plants when she studied with Don Elijio Panti, a 103-year-old Mayan H'men (shaman) in the great Mayan pyramids of Belize, Central America.

Take the time to plant a full-blown garden that will raise your level of health immeasurably, and treat your plants as if they were divine gifts. Food and healing herbs provide much more than the potential to provide nourishment. Their power is in direct proportion to the energy needed to survive by each plant. This why wild foods and herbs are all considered to have tremendous energy potential and vitality. Unfortunately, these wild plants are usually growing in an inappropriate place, generally causing them to be labeled as weeds.

Another problem is that domesticated vegetables and some fruits that we purchase from the grocery store have had their genetic makeup manipulated to create *big* fruits and vegetables. Strawberries are a good example. Wild strawberries are very small because they have their growth limitations imposed on them by genetics. This genetic information is stored in the nuclei of cells and dictates how much cell division (growth) will occur. However with DNA technology, scientists can manipulate the genetic code, and thereby increase the amount of cell division. This produces much larger fruits and vegetables than the natural evolutionary process provides for. Yes, the result is a larger and more plentiful harvest, but some of the concentrated energy potential has been sacrificed.

A Power Food: Bee Pollen
Bee pollen is considered one of nature's most completely nourishing foods, containing nearly all the nutrients required by human beings to sustain life. In his marvelous book, *Healing with Whole Herbs,* Paul

Pitchford describes it as food of the young bee that is a rich source of very digestible and usable protein, along with vitamin B-13.

In Chinese medicine, bee pollen is considered a tonic for energy and nutrition, and cultures throughout the world use it in a surprising number of applications: improving endurance and vitality, extending longevity, aiding in recovery from chronic illness, adding weight during convalescence, reducing cravings and addictions, regulating the intestines, and building new blood. Because it has antibiotic properties, it is also used to prevent communicable diseases such as the common cold and flu. Bee pollen is thought to protect against radiation and to possess cancer-preventative qualities. Pollen and raw unprocessed honey, which contains pollen, are remedies for many kinds of hay fever and allergies. And it can be given to children to help overcome retardation and other developmental problems.

The optimal dose of pollen varies with individual needs. For allergy prevention, for example, six grams daily in the form of tablets, capsules, or loose pellets (approximately one teaspoonful) is often sufficient. If you are taking it for hay fever, however, you must begin at least six weeks before hay-fever season begins and continue taking it throughout the season. Athletes seeking strength and endurance may ingest ten to fifteen grams or more daily.

Because bee pollen can cause extreme allergic reactions in some people, it is best to test for this possibility before taking a full dose. Start by taking just one pellet, and wait 15 to 20 minutes for allergic reactions such as coughing, breathing difficulties, or itching. A mild allergic reaction to any substance may be relieved by drinking one teaspoon of apple cider vinegar in one eight ounce glass of water at room temperature.

When taking bee pollen, be aware that the energy potential is incredible as opposed to those sugar-laden morning cereals we referred to earlier. It takes one bee, working eight hours a day for one month, to gather a six-gram dose. Each bee pollen pellet contains two million flower grains, and a teaspoonful contains 2.5 billion grains of flower pollen.[2]

Another Power Food: Dandelions

"Those darned dandelions!" Is this what your father used to say before he called the lawn service to annihilate those gorgeous yellow flowers in the spring? But the dandelion could save all those folks who severely compromise their health from the toxic chemicals sprayed on their lawns.

Dr. Rosita Arvigo[3] describes the *herb* (no, I don't refer to the dandelion as a "weed") as a liver cleanser. It also has the ability to raise low blood sugar was well as lower high blood sugar. Because the medicinal part of the plant is green, it contains calcium and chlorophyll, which makes it good muscle nutrition. Calcium and chlorophyll also purify the blood and stop the spread of bacteria, fungi, and other microorganisms.

Pick the leaves, after asking the plant's permission and thanking it for its healing properties, of course. The leaves are bitter (less so before the dandelion has bloomed and *very* bitter after), so try juicing fresh organic carrots with them to disguise the taste. Or, you can try Bubba Free John's suggestion for a green drink from his book, *The Eating Gorilla Comes in Peace:* Combine dandelions with several vegetables and herbal greens, such as beet tops, comfrey, and parsley, and process them in a blender with pineapple juice. This drink is high in trace minerals and vitamins and rejuvenates the whole body, especially the pancreas and liver.[4]

Nonetheless, the bitterness of the dandelion has a very important place in healing, making it a useful tool. Bitter foods and herbs drain various conditions associated with dampness, including lung congestion, candida yeast overgrowth, parasites, mucus, swellings, skin eruptions, abscesses, growths, tumors, cysts, and obesity. Bitter foods and herbs are also good for all moist accumulations, including edema in the regions governed by the spleen and pancreas (e.g., the intestines and the flesh of the body). Bitterness also increases intestinal muscle contractions[5], creating better elimination through the intestines.

My oldest polo pony provides an excellent example of the healing properties of the bitter dandelion. Pee Wee, who's approximately 23 years old, cannot eat any hay that has a speck of dust in it. Hay acquires dust if there is any moisture in the alfalfa, clover, or grasses at the time it is cut from the field and baled. The longer that tightly bound bale of hay sits, the greater the possibility that moisture will combine with the green plants and manufacture mold, producing a fine dust that makes Pee Wee so congested he labors to breathe.

This past year I took him to a new barn, gave him a nice warm stall, and checked the hay carefully. Within the first week, he had breathing problems. A little detective work and I discovered that the hay was being fed to him off the floor of the stall. Very dusty pine shavings covered the floor, and he was sucking up the dust with each mouthful of hay. Four days after I moved Pee Wee to an outdoors paddock, with good old *dirt*, he was breathing normally again. During those four days, he was allowed to munch on as many dandelions as he wanted.

So get out there and offer that unfortunate soul spraying the neighbor's lawn with insecticides a tantalizing dandelion cocktail!

More Power Foods: Micro-Algae—Spirulina, Chlorella, Blue-Green Algae

Micro-algae! Ever hear of them? They exist on the edge of the plant kingdom in that gray area between plant and animal. Algae are non-flowering water plants that grow in almost every drop of sunlit water, every grain of fertile soil, on the barks of trees, and the surfaces of rocks. "Oh, sounds delicious!" you say. "Let's go eat some lake scum!" But micro-algae are the most nutrient-dense of any natural food on the planet. These little powerhouses contain biologically active vitamins, minerals, trace elements, amino acids (for building protein), enzymes, fatty acids, and pigments such as the carotenoids and chlorophyll. In fact, micro-algae contain more chlorophyll than any other food (see chart for properties and actions of chlorophyll).

PROPERTIES AND ACTIONS OF CHLOROPHYLL

Purification	Anti-inflammation	Renewal
Stops bacterial growth in wounds, and anaerobic yeasts and fungi in the digestive tract	Counteracts the following inflammations: • sore throat • pyorrhea • gingivitis • stomach and intestinal inflammation and ulcers • all skin inflammations • arthritis pancreatitis	Builds blood Renews tissue Counteracts radiation Promotes healthful intestinal flora Improves liver function Activates enzymes to produce vitamins E, A, and K
Deodorizes: eliminates bad breath and body odor		
Removes drug deposits and counteracts all toxins; de-activates many carcinogens		
Halts tooth decay and gum infection (when used as a tooth powder)		

In their dried form (this is how you are likely to come into contact with these little gems), micro-algae contain the highest sources of protein, beta-carotene, and nucleic acids. Whether encapsulated or in a powdered drink that you mix with water, whether in the calcium-mineral formula I dispense in my office or straight from capsules found at the local health food store, micro-algae, such as spirulina, chlorella, and wild blue-green algae will improve your immune system and make your constitution stronger.

Spirulina can benefit those who eat an excess of animal protein, which does not assimilate well, and which burdens the body with waste products that are not properly excreted. These people are typically overweight, diabetic, hypoglycemic, cancerous, or arthritic:

> "By eating only 10-15 grams daily in this form (spirulina), the body normally becomes satisfied and animal protein is craved less. In addition, the severe liver damage resulting from malnutrition, alcoholism, or the consumption of nutrient-destroying food or drugs can be treated effectively by this type of nutrition. Spirulina also protects the kidneys against injury that occurs from taking strong prescription medication."[7]

Chlorella has a higher food value that spirulina but contains less protein and twice as much chlorophyll. It can be more expensive, though, because of the processing required to improve the digestibility of the tough outer cell wall. This cell wall binds heavy metals, pesticides, and such carcinogens as polychlorobiphenyls (PCB) and carries these toxins safely out of the body. Chlorella is considered the most toning of the micro-algae and the most gently cleansing. It is recommended for improving growth patterns in children, maintaining health in old age and healing injuries. It is also used to initiate growth where it has been stunted from disease or degenerative conditions, including Alzheimer's disease, sciatica, palsy, seizures, multiple sclerosis, nervousness, and other nerve disorders:

"Because its chlorophyll content is one of the highest of any food, chlorella is useful for the many conditions which benefit from chlorophyll's purification, renewal, and anti-inflammatory properties. Treatment of viruses and fungi which sap energy, such as candida yeast overgrowth, Epstein-Barr, chronic fatigue immune deficiency syndrome (CFIDS), and AIDS, is advanced by the immune-enhancing qualities of Chlorella Growth Factor as well as the antiviral effect of chlorophyll."[8]

While spirulina and chlorella are grown in a controlled medium, "wild blue-green grows naturally and was used by native peoples in Latin America and Africa for thousands of years, but there is no record of Native Americans using wild blue-green (Aphanizomenon)[9]." Today it is freeze-dried, which protects the algae from increased light and heat in the late summer which can transform it into an exceptionally toxic plant. William T. Barry, Northwest algae expert, limnologist, and professor at Gonzaga University in Spokane, Washington, claims that he has never found wild blue-green in its toxic state in Klamath Lake."

Its bitter flavor influences the "heart-mind" system. According to traditional Chinese medicine, bitter substances can focus the mind and improve concentration. Wild blue-green is also described as a mild diuretic, a neurostimulant, and an antidepressant. It is also excellent for the excessive, robust, overweight person or the depressed, flabby, person who has grown up with the modern diet of excessive meats, eggs, dairy, and rich, greasy, refined, chemical-ladened foods.

But micro-algae are not for everyone. People who are dry, thin, mentally unfocused, or sensitive, or those who have cold constitutions, will make their conditions worse if they ingest micro-algae. With extended use, other symptoms may include apathy, nonproductivity, lack of sexual desire and the beginning of an aching sensation in the lower back.[10]

The Real Thing

Hidden deep in the Prima Vera Forest outside of Guadalajara, Mexico, is the "Real Thing." No, it is not some rare herb or a precious gem. It is simply *water*—hot volcanic mineral water. No patient walks into my office without eventually getting a recommendation to soak in a bath rich in minerals. Sometimes that soothing bath has a cup or two of Masada bath salts, and sometimes it is enriched with Epsom Salts. More often I suggest mixing the two for economical reasons. But the Real Thing brings the healing power of Mother Nature into the picture once again.

Deep below the surface of a volcanic ridge one hour outside Guadalajara, inactive volcanoes represent the final stage of heat loss by igneous (crystalline rock) masses beneath the Earth's surface, which continue to give off vapors and gases while slowly cooling down. This gaseous phase is composed primarily of overheated steam that loses part of its heat while rising to the surface, where it expands and is transformed into hot-water (thermal) springs. However, almost all of the water discharged is surface water that penetrated deep into the Earth, encountered heat from volcanic magma (molten rock) and then quickly rose again to the surface.[11] This water contains mineral salts or gases usually classified as alkaline, saline, chalybeate (iron-containing), or sulfurous.[12]

When these mineral-bearing thermal waters of the Primavera Forest hit the surface, they emerge as the source of the Rio Caliente (Warm River), at a temperature of 157 degrees Fahrenheit. The Rio Caliente resort diverts part of the river (its waters have now cooled to 130 degrees) into four separate swimming pools and a steam sauna. Once a pool is filled, it takes about a day to naturally cool to between 100 and 97 degrees, then it is safe to indulge those sore, stiff joints and muscles. However, large red signs caution the guests to test the water temperature before entering the pools.

The soothing heat from this hot volcanic spring causes the pores of the skin to expand so that the precious variety of minerals from the water are easily absorbed. Dr. Dorothy Scuby[13] suggests that her patients drink a glass of distilled water about one half hour before a dunk in the pools. In distilled water, the H_2O molecule is devoid of any other molecular attachments, allowing it to draw needed minerals into the body. This process also works at home when you take a Masada or Epsom Salts bath.

Some of the visitors to Rio Caliente are senior citizens with stiffness and pain due to degenerating arthritic joints. Others, because of weak hearts and insufficient circulation, have trouble breathing, walking, or healing. In my case, a pulled hamstring muscle was strangling the nerves that run down the back of my leg, producing sciatic leg pain. My Valentine's Day present to myself was to finally get rid of the pain that radiated down my leg whenever I drove a car. So, I went to Rio Caliente to soak in the waters which, from the beginning of time, have been known for their healing properties.

Folks of all ages also come to the secluded spa to enjoy hiking in the Primavera Forest, where horses, donkeys, mules, and longhorn cattle roam wild. Three morning walks are provided, each at a different level of difficulty. Daily massages are available, as well as full-body mud packs and a vegetarian cuisine robust enough for any meat eater. My favorite pastime was horseback riding through terrain where Mexican bandit and revolutionary Pancho Villa hid out within viewing distance of the now famous Mt. Tequila, where most of the world's tequila is made.

Many hot mineral springs are not as accessible as Rio Caliente's beautiful resort with its clean, rectangular pools. In Hudspeth County south of El Paso along the Rio Grande, is a group of 22 natural pools that James A. Swan in his book, *Sacred Places*, describes as hard to find. The Indians felt these pools had sacred healing properties. Because each pool has a different mineral composition, each serves a specific function. For example, pools with the highest sulfur content are specifically used for cleansing the entire body, whereas others are used for diabetes or female complaints. The pools lie along continental fault lines, which means they are subject to electromagnetic field discharges.

Whether thermal hot springs are located at a luxurious resort or in rugged mountain terrain, it is always worth the climb, walk, or flight to find Mother Nature's healing baths. It always comes down to minerals. Essentially, you and I are merely mineral-rich sea water enclosed in a shell called the body. So, my best advice is to keep the mineral levels high, the range of motion as full as possible in every joint, and the water balance high enough to moisten all the body parts, and your perfect healing machine will operate to its fullest potential.

[1.] Depak Chopra.

[2.] Pitchford, pp. 111-112.

[3.] Rosita Arvigo, Lecture Chicago National College of Naprapathy, Chicago, IL. 1982.

[4.] Bubba Free John, *The Eating Gorilla Comes in Peace: The Transcendental Principle of Life Applied to Diet and the Regenerative Discipline of True Health* (The Down Horse Press, 1989), p. 554.

[5.] Pitchford, p. 274.

[6.] Pitchford, p. 188.

[7.] Pitchford, p. 191.

[8.] Pitchford, p. 193.

[9.] Pitchford, p. 194.

[10.] Pitchford, pp. 194-5.

[11.] *Encyclopedia Britannica*, 15th ed., "Volcanism," Vol. 29 (Encyclopedia Britannica, 1985), pp. 528-529.

[12.] *Encarta® 97 Encyclopedia*, "Mineral Water" (Microsoft® Corporation, 1993-1996).

[13.] Scuby, Personal conversation with Dr. Scuby summer 1997.

Chapter 8

Dr. Schmidt's Favorite Compresses

My Favorite Compress—the Palm of Christ

My favorite compress is made with castor oil. "Oh, no!" you say. "First she has us eating rabbit food. Then she takes away our soda pops. Now, she's trying to send us back to the Dark Ages where they poured castor oil down the throats of every poor kid who didn't do his or her duty at the outhouse three times a day." Well, you'll be happy to hear that castor oil (the Latin name is *Palma Christi*, meaning "the palm of Christ") is also used on the outside of the body as a compress.

Because castor oil has the ability to stimulate stagnated energy, I suggest using the compress on any muscular or skeletal strain or sprain that is not healing properly. I recommend its use on the joints of the knees and elbows. I also suggest it externally, over the top of any internal organ that's not working efficiently or any old surgery that's not healing the way it should. Castor oil does not just work right below the skin's surface, but has the ability to go very deep into the body's organs. It can be absorbed into the colon when we're constipated, into the liver when allergies are present, and into the female organs when we are experiencing any kind of female complaint. This compress is applied on the front of the body in the lower pelvis just below the navel. Castor oil sinks into the body and starts the energy flowing. It can even start the body healing an internal organ that has been in a chronically ill state. It has the ability to draw out and dissolve cysts, warts, growths, and other toxic accumulations. And it has an emollient effect that softens and removes scars.[1] Edgar Cayce even suggests applying a castor oil compress to heal cancerous tumors.

The compress consists of four layers (I repeat, four) of wool flannel, soaked with castor oil and laid over the problem area. One layer of plastic is placed on top of the flannel and then a heating pad (set on medium) or a hot water bottle is placed on top of the plastic. To make the compress, you need wool flannel—either an old wool flannel shirt or flannel you've bought from the fabric store. Cotton flannel will work, but wool is much better. Divide the material into four equal pieces, approximately one to two inches larger than the area you want to cover. Heat the oil slightly so it is warm to the touch, then soak the flannel with castor oil in a glass or plastic bowl.

Castor oil can be obtained at either a health food store or at most commercial drug stores. I recommend the health food store, because you may be able to obtain oil that has been cold-pressed, which works more efficiently than the kind processed with heat (usually found at drug stores).

To gain the correct stimulating effects, place the compress over the affected area for one hour each day. After compressing for an hour, simply place the flannel in the bowl, cover it with the plastic and shove it out of the way. The compress can be used repeatedly for one week without changing the flannel, occasionally adding a little more oil.

In my practice, I have recommended that the caster oil compress be applied on the liver, specifically for increasing the brain's ability to absorb information. A patient's eight-grade son was having difficulty keeping his grades up, so a compress was applied to his liver late each evening. The liver's circadian rhythm is highest between 8 and 9 P.M.—the natural time of day that it begins cleaning the body. (Imagine the maid coming in and cleaning house quietly while you sleep.) How wonderful to awake to a body that neatly arranged all the toxins while you rested. All you need do is simply take out the "garbage" with each morning's bowel movement.

The patient applied the compress to her son's liver for an hour each evening for two weeks. Two months later she reported that his teachers wanted to know what had happened to her son. Had he taken a special learning course? Had he gotten a tutor? His grades and his attitude had improved immensely.

I have also suggested a castor oil compress to prevent a root canal. Jane had been bothered with recurring tooth pain from one of her upper molars for about one month before she consulted her dentist, who recommended that she have a root canal. Though the X-rays showed no bone deterioration at the base of the tooth, her dentist felt a root canal would eventually be the answer. Then Jane asked what I might recommend, and I explained to her that the base of the tooth is like any other part of the body that needs a steady circulation of blood, vital energy and a clear path along which to remove debris from the inflammation.

The glands under the arms, just under the ears, under the muscles of the cheeks, and the sinuses behind the facial bones are the pathways that should carry away any inflammation that lies beneath a troubled tooth. I imagine all these points as balloons full with the products of the inflammation being generated at the base of the tooth. Each full balloon crowds all the other tissues that surround it—tissues filled with nerve fibers that become very angry about this crowding. That's why the tooth sends such loud pain signals. But if each balloon had a chance to drain, then the tissues under the tooth could receive fresh blood, vital nutrients to fight infection, and would not be so engorged that pain receptors are sparked each time a breath is taken. If given the opportunity, the body does an amazing job of healing itself.

With that simple explanation of how her lymphatic drainage system works, Jane was able to speed the healing process along herself. I showed her how to rub the surface of the skin just over each one of the glands for one or two minutes, starting under her arm, working her way up to the ear, and, finally, over the sinuses in her face. Then I instructed her to make a castor oil compress to cover the tooth, her ear, and part of her neck. Jane compressed for one hour at the end of each day, after first massaging her glands. Then she rubbed Tea Tree Oil into the gums surrounding the inflamed tooth—initially every fifteen minutes for a two-hour period, and then, four times a day. Three days later she was pain free and never had a problem with the tooth again.

A few words of caution: Because it can induce miscarriages, castor oil is *not* recommended during pregnancy. Also, because the oil is thick and messy, I suggest that you put towels underneath yourself to keep from dripping oil on your bedding. However, the amazing benefits of this stimulating natural compress are worth the small mess. Several hours after using the castor oil compress, your skin will feel softer than it has in years. Try coating those dry feet twice a week and see the wonderful change.

My Second Favorite Compress—Comfrey Root

Tim worked part-time as a sign painter, and in his free time he was an avid Ultimate Frisbee™ athlete. Ultimate is played like soccer, but players use a Frisbee™ instead of a ball. There's a lot of jumping in the air, wild catches, and crashing into bodies—all without the protection of any upper-body padding, only shin guards. By the end of each game, players can be bruised and banged from head to toe, and Tim was no exception. He came to me several times to treat his discolored, disjointed, and out of shape body. Although the naprapathic-chiropractic treatments worked wonderfully, Tim also wanted something to prevent inflammation on the field, where his injuries occurred. We used two different products.

The first was comfrey root, one of my favorite anti-inflammatory herbs. I instructed Tim to make a compress to apply topically over any injury he received while playing. I suggested using two to three teaspoons of the powdered comfrey, or six or seven capsules broken apart, spread on a clean cotton wash cloth that had been folded in half. The powdered-herb area should be approximately one half inch larger than the area of the bump, bruise, or in extreme cases, broken bone.

Secondly, I suggested that Tim spray Zheng Gu Shui liniment directly on his skin and on the comfrey root compress as well. The alcohol in the liniment breaks down the herb's properties so they can pass into the body. Because the liniment contains a combination of Chinese herbs, menthol, cinnamon, and camphor, it acts as a stimulant that encourages the body to absorb herbs quickly.

If Tim were to use this compress at home, I would suggest that the powder be broken down with approximately one-quarter cup of boiling water, drizzled over comfrey that has been spread on a cotton dish cloth. As boiling water is drizzled over the herb, a knife or spoon is used to mix the water and comfrey into a paste. Then the injury site should be lightly misted with Zheng Gu Shui, and covered with the pasty compress.

I stress the fact that the cloth should not be soaking wet, only moistened. This compress is very cooling and will remove any hot inflammation from swollen ankles or knees with amazing swiftness. A sopping wet cloth will only lower the skin's temperature even more, which can chill the patient in cool weather.

[1.] Pitchford, p. 146.

Chapter 9

Favorite Chinese Remedies

Chinese Tea and Rabbit Turds

I have already mentioned that the wonderful, sometimes life-saving herbal teas that my Chinese physician and mentor used to give me for various health reasons tasted awful. No, that's not quite accurate. They tasted worse than awful! Well, at least mine did. Those liver-cleansing, fire-reducing teas were bitter, while the teas to strengthen the heart tended to be more on the sweet side. The teas prescribed for children had a much milder taste, and their dose was a couple of ounces.

Within the last few years, the herbs have been compressed into round, black or dark brown pellets, affectionately known as "rabbit turds" around my office. It's much easier to swallow ten to fifteen of these compressed herbs than one cup of the doctor's tea concoctions, and my patient compliance has risen about 99 percent since the pellets were introduced. These pellets come in formulas for heart and blood circulation, problems with the female organs (from PMS to infertility), kidneys, diabetes, fat reduction, beauty, and even one for children's growth and better overall health.

Facial Diagnoses—Everything Is More Than it Seems

Facial diagnosis is an important component of the Chinese medical procedure. When evaluating which formula to recommend, Dr. Lau takes a good long look at a patient's face, examining the forehead, eyes, cheeks, ears, and the area around the mouth. [**Figure 9.1**]

The ears reflect the entire body. Actually, the bottom of the ear corresponds to the top of the body, while the top of the ear corresponds to the bottom of the body.

The forehead, or more particularly, the triangular area just above the nose, reflects the health of the liver. The top of the forehead correlates to systemic energy, or the vitality of our entire system. The area just above the eyes and the eyelids (which women love to cover with exotic shades of color created from chemicals and heavy metals) reflect the female organs—the ovaries and uterus. The next time you have the urge to paint your eyes, remember that you are essentially stuffing your uterus with toxic metals.

The cheeks reveal the energy coming from the lungs. Discoloration may indicate irregularities in the lining of the lungs—an unhappy thought if you are a smoker. The area directly underneath the eyes reflects kidney energy. Someone approaching death, whose energy is drained (the kidneys hold vital energy for life), will have dark puffy circles underneath their eyes. Allergies to certain foods, especially those foods that the unsuspecting individual eats every day, puts the adrenal glands into constant emergency alert, depleting their energy. Because these glands sit atop the kidneys, dark under-eye circles can also indicate the presence of an allergy. In addition, patients who drink several cups of coffee a day reflect that stress to the kidneys with dark circles under their eyes.

The area around the mouth, specifically the lips, corresponds to the stomach and the digestive system. This is where Dr. Lau begins

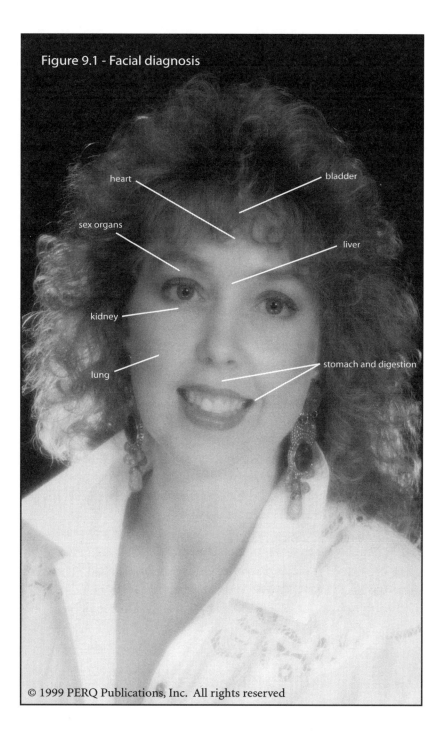

Figure 9.1 - Facial diagnosis

heart

bladder

sex organs

liver

kidney

lung

stomach and digestion

when he makes his facial diagnosis. Have you ever wondered why some children lick their lips? It is because they are trying to put a coat of moisture over very uncomfortably chapped skin. I've also seen adults unwittingly try to do the same thing. Because the lips reflect the health of the stomach and its ability to digest, chapped lips indicate a problem with digestion. Thus, people can be observed licking their lips after eating meat or dairy, or applying lipstick or lip balm to relieve the discomfort.

With children, I usually suspect a dairy allergy. With adults, I suspect that they are not able to digest large heavy protein meals of beef, pork, or lamb. But always, I am amazed at the phenomenal ability of the body to develop mechanisms that let us know (long before the existence of diabetes, heart disease—or other major disease conditions are diagnosed) that we are not processing our meats nor assimilating our fats, and are having a problem transforming our food into available energy. The body uses facial language to shout out loud that something is wrong. But again and again, lipstick is applied to alleviate the symptom, with no understanding of what the body is communicating. A child that consistently breaks out around the mouth and chin is having difficulty digesting properly and dairy products should be eliminated from their diet. Cold sores or fever blisters indicate that the stomach is nervous and upset. Large doses of my herbal calcium have a soothing and calming effect on the stomach, while coffee, cheese, spicy, and greasy foods will further irritate the stomach.

What can you do? First make a record of the foods that you've eaten that seem to cause your lips to become uncomfortable. Be observant. Be with your body. Then you can apply no. 1 or no. 2 Chinese cream to help heal your sore chapped lips. no. 1 has no taste at all, so it will not be offensive to children (though no. 2 has a taste that children will say is terrible).

No. 1 and No. 2 Chinese Creams
Through my favorite Chinatown healers, Dr. Pak Lau and his daughter, Dr. Lisa, I discovered two wonderful healing creams,

simply named no. 1 and no. 2. Because the sequence in which they are applied is no. 2 first and no. 1 second (how confusing), I'll begin by telling you about no. 2.

No. 2 cream, which is made from crushed pearls, is both an anti-inflammatory and antiseptic ointment with remarkable pain-killing properties. As my daughter, who has been raised exclusively on this amazing take-the-pain-away-in-30-seconds treatment, says, "It's made with magic, Mom!" For child or adult, whether the injury is a smashed finger, scraped knee, bee sting, cut, or laceration, I recommend no. 2 cream—no more stinging Bactine® on those injuries. This thin white ointment should be applied immediately when the injury occurs, and because of its fast absorption quality, the body will suck it right in. As soon as that happens, usually within three to five minutes, apply some more. Its wonderful pain-killing quality takes hold almost immediately.

Late one Sunday night, Sandy called me. Four of her six children had been wrestling on the bed, and one of her sons was injured. She was sure he had a broken finger. She brought him to my house that same evening (if I had been in my office, I would have pulled out my trusty tuning fork, slapped it on my palm and then placed it on the supposed broken bone—a fractured bone becomes more painful when the vibrations from the tuning fork shake it). The boy's finger could bend slightly, but it was starting to swell, and I felt an X-ray was needed. In the meantime, I covered it with a thick layer of no. 2 cream, and within three or four minutes, the pain seemed to disappear and the swelling never increased after that point. Sandy continued to apply the cream a couple of times throughout the night until the finger could be X-rayed first thing in the morning. It was then discovered that the boy had a hairline fracture. The doctor wiped the no. 2 cream off and applied a splint. Ten or fifteen minutes after the cream was removed, the boy began to complain of pain for the first time.

No. 2 cream is also good for rashes, psoriasis, or any kind of itching from any source, including diaper rash. But you must remember that the skin is our largest organ, and has an important part to play in our overall health. The skin can remove cellular waste and toxic substances very swiftly by pushing them out through the pores. If someone suffers from persistent rashes, not necessarily due to contact with a poisonous plant, the colon's health and the body's elimination system must be examined to ascertain if the skin is taking over the colon's job of kicking out poisons. If this is the case, no. 2 cream is applied only *after* very warm water treatments to the affected skin. If no. 2 cream is applied to an area of skin that is still attempting to spit out toxic waste materials, the cream often traps the toxins inside the skin, and the body will only itch more.

The body makes us itch for a specific reason. When we itch, we scratch and flood the area with blood. This increases circulation so that the offending toxic elements can be carried away by the increased blood flow. If we scratch until we actually break the outer layer of skin, we allow the toxic elements to escape. Think of this toxic component as heat. It carries all the components of heat such as redness and swelling (the skin is actually hot to the touch). Scratching opens up the pores and allows the heat to leave the body through the broken skin.

Instead of scratching, place the body part that itches under a faucet of warm water. Slowly raise the water's temperature to promote the itch, but be careful not to burn the skin. As the temperature is raised, the skin itches more and more until, after several minutes, there's no itch left. The heat element that the Chinese recognize as causing itch has left the body through the skin's expanded pores. At this point, it is safe to apply the no. 2 cream. If it is put on prematurely, the body, in its infinite wisdom, will make the skin itch even more. Or, the toxic heat component may travel to another area of the body where it will make itself known.

Because the liver processes toxic waste materials, it can suffer further symptoms if the heat is not expelled from the body. The next logical step is to check the Chinese chart of hot and cold foods to see if you are eating too many hot, dry, spicy, or peppery substances. The objective is to be in balance. Some foods have cooling properties, and some have heating properties. A diet that is primarily one or the other is out of balance and will create the perfect environment for disease to cultivate.

No. 1 cream is an ancient healing formula composed primarily of the herb gypsum, and is used for cuts, scrapes, bruises, broken bones, facial acne, and cold sores. I have used it on my own broken bones and have witnessed a speedy healing process. However, to alleviate the pain and inflammation of the initial injury, start with no. 2 cream. After 24 hours, switch to the no. 1 cream, which works nicely to bring the healing elements to the site of the wound. It is a thick, waxy, topical substance that, unlike no. 2 cream, is not completely absorbed by the skin but stays on the surface. It can be applied generously, with the area then wrapped lightly with gauze so that the cream is not rubbed off by clothing.

I have also found no. 1 cream to be very effective for old surgeries that have not healed. For instance, bunion surgery can often solve foot problems of excessive bone growth, but occasionally I see patients who are thinking about having it redone because of the continual pain at the site where the bunion was removed. I suggest that they first apply no. 1 cream, massaging it in thoroughly, and then spray Zheng Gu Shui liniment over the cream. The cream is the healing element, while the liniment is the stimulant that drives the cream into the body so that the old surgery can mend. The cream needs to be applied two to three times daily for at least one to three months, depending on the rate of healing.

In the case of chronic low-back pain, where X-rays have determined that arthritis, bone degeneration, or disc narrowing is present, I use no. 1 cream to make the patient more comfortable. I have several senior patients with arthritic spurring in the neck or arthritic joints in the low back. I suggest that they rub the cream in vigorously, like a two-minute massage, on a daily basis. When finished with the massage, they are to apply a thick layer of cream and then put on a T-shirt so that their outer clothing does not absorb it.

I've never seen X-rays to support the contention that the bone is repaired, but patients report that they are more pain-free and better able to turn and bend forward. Several of my senior patients use no. 1 cream every day on stiff immovable necks, where arthritis has limited their ability to turn and look behind them.

Kidney (or Vital) Energy, Fear, Hair Loss, and Snakes

The Chinese regard the kidneys as the organ in charge of the essential energy in the body. As I've already mentioned, with facial diagnosis, the health of the kidneys can be ascertained by examining the area immediately under the eyes. When someone is just about to pass away (or pass over), we might notice that the skin underneath the eyes is gray and there is puffiness or large swollen bags. As the energy of life drains away, so the natural coloration of the face just below the eyes drains to the color of ashen gray. Coffee dehydrates and stresses the kidneys. It is essential to cut back on or eliminate coffee when trying to reach a more optimal state of health.

Another characteristic of depleted kidney energy in women is thinning hair. Hair that falls out in handfuls is not very typical of women. In males, it may have to do with genetics, but in women it has more to do with kidney energy. According to both Western and Eastern studies of the body and its functions, the kidneys balance and maintain the body's fluids. When the kidney system is weakened and the kidneys out of balance, the flow of nutrients through the blood system to bones, ears, hair follicles, urinary tract, and bladder are also out of balance. With limited energy, fluids barely reach the outer extremities. The scalp is an outer extremity. When not enough blood reaches the hair, the hair follicles aren't being enriched with enough moisture to keep them alive. In women, this can cause their hair to fall out.

"Out of balance" is a simple phrase but it can mean that a combination of factors is contributing to kidney weakness. Staying up late can tax the kidney's vital energy. Working long hours, ice cold drinks, and an excessive amount of orgasms (unfortunately, for some) can also drain precious kidney energy. General symptoms, including all bone problems—especially those of the knees, lower back, and teeth; hearing loss and ear infections; head-hair problems such as hair loss, split ends, and premature graying; any urinary, sexual, or reproductive imbalances; or poor growth and development of the mind and body, including premature aging—can all be an indication of kidney imbalance.[1]

Fear is the emotion held in the kidneys. While a little healthy fear often protects us, excessive, deeply rooted fear and insecurity can injure the kidneys. Pitchford suggests that "the fear-ridden kidney (Water Element) fails to remove the excessive water, which extinguishes the heart spirit (Fire Element) and its normal expression of love and joy."[2] I can't tell women experiencing hair loss what they fear; they must listen to their own bodies in quiet contemplation and realize their fear themselves. I can only relate how my own experience with fear influenced my personal healing evolution.

We have an old cistern on our farm that seems to be a breeding ground for garden snakes. We also let the grass in the front of the house grow long so that our horses can "mow" the lawn. These factors, plus the fact that I'm afraid of snakes, make all the snakes in the area love our property. I don't like snakes, but I believe in live and let live, so I was determined to just let them be because they are also sacred creatures of the Great Spirit.

I never seem to see a snake until I'm about to step on one, and it darts away with lightning speed. Then I let out a blood-curdling scream and start crying. It happens every time, whether I want it to or not. I was sure that this fear started at the age of five. I distinctly remembered walking into a crowd of children on the school playground and accidentally stepping on a snake they were staring at in amazement. It scared me to death, and I cried then, too.

As an adult, I found the courage to pick snakes up on the end of my pitchfork and toss them across the street. But a friend who lives on a hunting resort reported that researchers had taken a very large snake two miles from its original habitat and put a tracking device on it, only to have it travel right back in one day's time. So, my next scheme was to put them into a five-gallon bucket, and cover it with a wooden board and a rock while I transported them out of town about five miles away from our farm.

One particularly beautiful June afternoon, all that changed. I had saddled my favorite horse Pee Wee and started out the driveway. Hondo, a man I lived with on the farm, was removing the last pieces of a dead tree from in front of the house. Suddenly, he held a large chunk of wood from the tree over his head and smashed it down onto the street. Then he picked up another chunk and again hurled it down. As I drew closer, I discovered that he was acting so curiously because he was trying to kill a medium-size snake that was in the middle of the road angrily rattling its tail at him. It was a timber rattler, which I had never before seen in our gardens. This is where I drew the line. We had children running all through those lawns, and enough was enough. I began killing all the garden snakes I encountered by chopping off their heads with a shovel. This was not done in anger but only out of tremendous fear.

As always, when I'm facing a difficult situation like this, Lee, one of my most enlightened patients, needed a naprapathic treatment for her back. Whenever I have a problem, or I'm stuck on an issue, she seems to need a treatment. I learn so much from my patients like Lee that I should be paying *them* for the counseling.

"Behavior patterns can stem from fears held for a long time. Sometimes longer than our present memories," she said. "There's more than meets the eye here with all these snakes." She then recommended that I undergo some hypnosis to discover why.

I went to see Janet, my hypnotherapist, who gently and calmly relaxed me by having me count backward from one hundred. At ninety-six, when all the numbers disappeared, she instructed me to notice each body part and to let go of the tension held there until my concentration was pinpointed on her every word. When I refer patients to Janet, I tell them not to worry about the question of past memories or past lives if their religious beliefs did not accept this concept. Imagine that you are merely working with a metaphoric memory brought up by the subconscious to create a better understanding of a pressing issue in this world.

I traveled back from the present, past the snake incident in the schoolyard, to another lifetime in which I saw myself as a four-year-old child in India. We were poor farmers, and I was out with my father as he worked the fields. But he wasn't keeping an eye on me, and I wandered out into the tall grasses and was swallowed whole by an enormous snake. Reliving my death as the huge viper coiled itself more tightly around me, crushing the breath out of my small frail body, was terrifying. I screamed and wept. I was hovering over the scene as an observer and, at the same time, I was in the scene as a participant, actually re-experiencing the initial pain and horror. A trained hypnotherapist can help you clear these terrible past-life traumas by making you participant and observer simultaneously. In this manner, some of the tremendous pain is more easily experienced.

With Janet reassuringly by my side, I was able to explore and question the remembrance. I discovered that the Indian father was actually Hondo. Just like the Indian father of my past life, he is quite busy, and there are no tight-knit partnership qualities in our relationship. As Janet questioned me further, I admitted that if any man I was romantically involved with became too assertive, too possessive, too smothering, I wanted out fast.

"Did you hear what you said?" Janet exclaimed. "You just recalled a past-life death in which you were smothered by a huge snake, and now in this life you can't stand to be smothered in any manner by the affection of men that you're in relationships with!" The cool wind of spiritual truth gave me goose bumps all over. Of course, she was right! I never could have seen the correlation between the two myself. But as she said it, it felt perfect.

According to the Chinese calendar, I was born in the year of the snake. Whether or not this is a coincidence, I don't know; however, I now understand that I need to thank all the snakes that have crossed my path, and to ask forgiveness of the ones whose lives I've taken. Although I have not yet picked one up (but I'm going to), I did actually touch a large snake at the pet fair at my daughter's school this spring.

I strongly suggest that you examine your own rigid beliefs, fears, and compulsive behavior patterns through the use of hypnosis, for they may be more than they appear on the surface. The beauty of this system is that once those behavior patterns are discovered, unearthed, and understood, you can move beyond them. Native Americans say that snakes bring wisdom, which is certainly true in my case. Through my experience with snakes, I can now move to a relationship that is nurturing, without always feeling smothered. I am growing.

---

[1] Pitchford, p. 316.

[2] Ibid.

Chapter 10

Naprapathic History

I am a naprapath, and the treatment I give is mostly naprapathic. However, I am also a chiropractor—not by choice, but simply because of a hard nudge from the state of Illinois. One day, I was a practicing naprapath, operating under Illinois's drugless practitioner classification. The next, after a change in the law concerning the practice of medicine in the state, I would suddenly be considered a felon for touching and giving medical treatments to the spine. Of course, the newly revised law stated that chiropractors, osteopaths, and MDs could practice naprapathy, despite the fact that none of these groups knows anything about the practice or cares to know. But for naprapaths, the only recourse was to become MDs, chiropractors, or osteopaths. Okay, I couldn't fight city hall or the State of Illinois, so I went for a chiropractic degree in order to do what I had already been doing for six years.

But, let me start at the beginning. In 1982 when I began my study of naprapathy, Dr. Roland Sidney ran the naprapathic college. He was a large man with an equally large grin. He believed wholeheartedly in naprapathy and worked very hard to promote this small profession. He had his own private practice, seeing patients as they arrived at his office rather than by appointment. Thus, he often worked very late into the evening, past 11 P.M. Yet, he also found time to educate, teaching a course at the college called "The Essence of Naprapathy." And he was entrusted with the care and development of each crop of budding new students that arrived at the school.

These students came to Dr. Sidney having been influenced by a lifetime of medical care, overseen by traditional AMA doctors who had guided them through flu, measles, injections, and tonsillectomies. By studying naprapathy, they were walking away from their faithful doctors and into the blasphemy of alternative holistic healing. Dr. Sidney introduced them to a world of healing that considers the body a perfect healing machine. He introduced them to a world where cold symptoms are not stopped, fever is considered an ally, and where a twice yearly occurrence of hay fever is merely an announcement of how filthy a body's system is. In other words, Dr. Sidney blew their concept of healing into a thousand pieces.

During class, he would tell story after amazing story about his patients. For example, one man had an amputated leg, but still had phantom pains that ran up and down his hip into the missing limb. The whole class listened in awe as Dr. Sidney described inserting acupuncture needles into the acupuncture points that no longer existed on the missing limb, mysteriously relieving the man's pain.

He spoke of "sandwiches" (one of his favorite phrases) and how parasites, bacteria, and viruses won't stay in a body unless there are sandwiches (i.e., waste products and unwanted debris) to eat. These invaders come into the body and pick up the debris and waste, and when it is all gone, they leave. In other words, we are nothing but a free meal for bugs. Of course, he was alluding to poisons and cellular waste materials that don't belong in our systems. Invading bacteria and viruses exist in those systems as allies, pick up the debris, devour the waste, and encourage the body's defense mechanisms to begin the cleanup process. With this little bit of spring cleaning, the amazing self-healing body is running efficiently once more. Dr. Sidney was a very good friend of Dr. Norman Esserman, who was both a lawyer and a naprapath. Although he didn't practice naprapathy professionally, he told me that he thought naprapathy was as close to the truth as a healing profession could be, and he wanted to be a part of it.

One year, he came to the naprapathic convention with tremendous gallbladder pain. He was thin, his color was very gray, and his cheeks shallow. I had seen dozens of people at the college with aches, pains, bad backs, and stiff necks, but I had never seen anyone who looked like their vital life force was draining away before my very eyes. But that's what Dr. Esserman looked like, and everyone could tell he was extremely ill.

He and Dr. Sidney had always thought of me as special. I delivered goat's milk and cheeses and freshly baked breads every Thursday afternoon from a farm near my horses, and both of them always looked forward to my organic delivery. When they boarded the elevator for Dr. Esserman's room, they invited me along. Because I was a new student and curious to see what one would actually do with a really sick person, I followed along like a hypnotized puppy.

Dr. Esserman stretched out on the hotel bed, and Dr. Sidney began to do some very deep pulling, twisting and massage-like strokes in the area of the gallbladder in order to drain the liver and gallbladder of their toxic accumulations. Dr. Esserman burped and belched and burped again. The gas that came out of that man was incredible and smelled terrible from both ends. I thought for sure that at any moment an ambulance was going to come and carry this poor soul away. Dr. Sidney was getting right down into the core of this man's abdominal cavity. He was stretching, pulling and digging so deeply that I was amazed that a stomach was that pliable.

After the treatment, Dr. Esserman got up and wearily took the elevator down to another session of the convention. A couple of hours later, both men returned to the room, and I tagged along again.

Dr. Esserman looked terrible, and he looked tired. He was physically drained. But Dr. Sidney continued to work on him several times—and he continued to belch and burp. What Dr. Sidney was performing was a liver, gallbladder, colon manipulation to dislodge toxic accumulations from these organs and then gently guide them through the natural course of the colon. By the third day of the convention, Dr. Esserman began to look better. Color returned to his cheeks and he started to eat once more. By the time I saw him again in class, he was back to his old self.

I was amazed and in awe. I felt as though I had walked into the world's biggest secret. I had been allowed to enter the relatively unknown society of natural healers that was privy to mysteries and truths the AMA had never imagined, let alone questioned. I wondered why the profession—this center of the universe of medical healing—had stayed so small. Why hadn't it grown? Why hadn't it spread, in the United States, beyond the state of Illinois? Why hadn't these marvelous healers given this profession to the world?

Twelve years later, I understand the yin and yang of things. I understand that the profession needed to go through its due share of political turmoil, and that issues of licensure for a healing art that had been around since 1908 needed to stagnate in the state legislature in order to push me into becoming a chiropractor. Although I am still not considered to be a "real medical doctor," people will come to see you if you are a real healer, no matter what your title. I choose to use the naprapathic treatments on my patients, sprinkling in the in-depth education I received as a chiropractic.

I wanted to be a naprapath because I had known a naprapath, had been helped by naprapathic treatments, and thought it was a good and worthwhile profession. Sounds good. Sounds noble. But wait until I get into the politics of it.

Naprapathy is an offshoot of the chiropractic profession and has been around since 1908, when chiropractors split into different factions as a result of differences in opinion as to the fundamental cause of disease in the human body. Naprapathy's founder was Dr. Oakley Smith, a "one-time Iowa medical student who had investigated Andrew Still's osteopathy in Kirksville, Missouri before going to Davenport to first become a chiropractor." He would reject in time the Palmer chiropractic concept of vertebral subluxation in favor of the "connective tissue doctrine of disease".[1] He was convinced that pathology to the connecting tissues, espe-

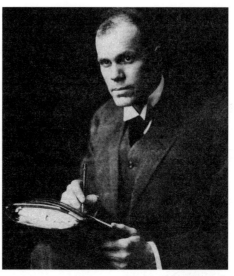

Dr. Oakley Smith
"The Father of Naprapathy"

cially ligaments, "almost invariably undergoes a permanent change as a result of a temporary injury."[2] That chronic or permanent abnormal change which can influence nerve transmission, was his underlying theory to the cause of most human ailments. Dr. Smith published a Connective Monograph in 1919 in which he said:

> "Whenever nerves, blood vessels, or lymphatics are surrounded and protected by connective tissue whose fibers are arranged in such a way that the common accidents of the body may bring undue strain upon them, a consequent alteration in the length of the structures which these fibers compose will alter the tension upon such nerves and vessels and will weakend or irritate them. An irritated or weaken nerve invariably means abnormal action or disease of the structures which that nerve supplies. An impediment to the flow of blood or lymph also means perverted action, the extent of which depends upon the structures disturbed."[3]

Prior to the creation of naprapathy, Dr. Smith traveled to Germany and Czechoslovakia in 1890, exploring ancient healing practices of manipulation and massage techniques. Dr. George Goetschel, a chiropractor whose father was a naprapath and one of Oakley's best friends, told me how he had been entranced with Oakley's tales of different healing methods, including trained bears who walked on people's achy backs in Eastern Europe. In Czechoslovakia, Oakley learned a "rough" (meaning rustic or basic) massage technique called Napravit (which means "to fix"), with which he combined with his knowledge of chiropractic bone adjustment.

Upon his return in 1900 and until 1911, the State of Illinois made available a registry that separated medical doctors from other physicians. Dr. Oakley Smith was second in line in the Office of the Illinois Secretary of State to register for this new certificate of licensure on June 16, 1904, as a chiropractor. Dr. Minora Paxson stood just in front of Oakley and is identified as holding the first certificate in Illinois licensing a woman chiropractor, as well as being the first licensed chiropractor in the world. This new designation as an Other Practitioner (OP) included dentists, chiropractors, optometrists, and pharmacists. But it was not until August 3, 1908, that Dr. Smith coined the word "naprapathy." By September 30 of the same year, he had incorporated his not-for-profit college,[4] he was granted this corporate status from the state to confer degrees in the newly formed, drugless health profession called naprapathy. His school was the only one of its kind. In 1912, the school underwent a corporate name change to the Chicago School of Naprapathy.

Those who knew Dr. Oakley personally said he was an intellectual, and after his first anatomy course at the University of Davenport, he was fascinated with the engineering of the spine. He has also been described as outspoken and domineering, and he considered naprapathy his cherished baby. No one was going to tell him how to run the show.

But it is the state's job to set the guidelines for medical professionals. The State of Illinois and the Department of Records and Education in June of 1917 put together those guidelines of practicing medicine in the Medical Practice Act. They established the distinction that exists today, dividing health practitioners into the two classifications of those dispensing medicine, drugs, and performing surgery, and those that are drugless healers with no invasive surgery. But a vague area of contention existed within this act that stated that a healer, osteopath, or chiropractor that studied "any system or method of treating human ailments" also required a license. This new form of a license, though available to the osteopath and chiropractor, was not for the naprapath. This act also tried to restrict and limit the chiropractic profession by exercising its proper use of the police power of the state by fixing the educational standards and requiring that a chiropractor be in good standing and repute when graduating from a four-year course of instruction. There was no chiropractic school or college in the country that had a four-year course of study, and the resulting court action in June of 1921 reversed sections of this Medical Practice Act as unconstitutional on the grounds that no other school or college had more than a two-year course beyond common school and high school. The judgment summarized with the statement that "Surely, then, there is no reason for providing that the limited professional education of one class of physicians shall be greater or for a longer time than that for those practicing medicine and surgery in all their branches.[5]" While declaring this section of the Medical Practice Act unconstitutional and unjustly discriminating,[6] also found it arbitrary and unreasonable for chiropractors to be required to secure recommendations of moral and professional character from two medical men or osteopathic physicians. When the judgment was reversed the court said:

> "The prejudice existing against chiropractors by medical men or osteopathic physicians is known to be intense and in many cases very unreasonable. For a chiropractor to have to conform to such a regulation would in all probability result in his being excluded from any examination whatever by reason of his inability to obtain such a certificate, although

he might be able to establish a good moral character
and a good professional standing by good, compe-
tent men in his own or other professions or callings
outside of the medical profession."[7]

Several times the State Of Illinois, spurred on by the Department
of Records and Education and their sacred need "to protect the
people against ignorance, incapacity, deception, or fraud in the practice of the medical profession"[8], charged naprapaths with practicing
medicine without a license. In one landmark case in 1924, _People
v. Witte_, Dr. Smith hired renowned lawyer Clarence Darrow—the
defense attorney in the famous Scopes "monkey" trial—to test the
constitutionality of this 1917 Medical Practice Act just as the chiropractic profession has done. Dr. Edwin F. Witte claimed to be a valid
healing professional, having graduated from the naprapathic college,
but was unable to obtain a license from the state. Oakley's naprapathic curriculum lacked the diversified science program similar
to the chiropractic program, which was a criteria the state demanded
for a licensure program. Attorney Darrow's client, Dr. Witte, was
found guilty of practicing medicine without a license.[9]

In 1926 another naprapath, Dr. Barnett, was convicted of engaging
in the treatment of human ailments without a license. Upon
appeal, the defendant conceded that he did not have a license but
argued that the Act did not provide for licensure of naprapaths.
The court rejected the defendant's argument and held, after
reviewing the Act, that there was ample provision under the law
for the examination and licensure of those desiring to practice
naprapathy.[10]

Conversations with older naprapaths raised the issue of education.
The chiropractic education included many of the basic science
studies. Dr. Smith maintained through the troubled political years
that the healing practice of naprapathy was scientifically intact,
complete, and a tremendous healing system needing no additional
studies, and he was not going to be forced into adding those
sciences, either. So, the profession went into the years of turmoil.

The State of Illinois again took legal action when, in 1938, Charlotte Hermes, an investigator for the Department of Registration and Education of the State of Illinois, presented herself to Dr. W. J. Elmore as Mrs. Ralph Sigmund and said that she had been referred to him by her sister-in-law, who lived on 59th Street. She told Dr. Elmore that she was suffering from severe headaches, pains in the back of her eyes, and pains in the arms and shoulders. Dr. Elmore examined her spine and the location of sore spots; told her she would need a course of treatments which would cost $12. Dr. Elmore suggested that she take six treatments and the diagnosis would be free, but that if she took no further treatments, the diagnosis would be $5. Charlotte Hermes testified that she called again on the following June 2nd, and that Dr. Elmore examined her back and neck by pressing on the vertebra; that he informed her that the pains in her shoulders and arms were caused by pinched nerves, and explained that a chiropractor would consider it a "subluxation". Dr. Elmore applied pressure to the witness's back and to her neck and shoulders. He also gave her a treatment with a machine to which there were rubber pads connected; Dr. Elmore put one pad on Charlotte Hermes's back and the other to her right side. She experienced considerable heat for about twenty minutes and that he manipulated her neck and shoulders. He also removed her shoes and gave her feet a similar treatment. For this treatment, the witness testified that she paid him $5.

The Court of Cook County in Illinois, Justices Hebel and Sullivan concurred that the defendant, Dr. Elmore was guilty of engaging in the diagnosis and treatment of ailments of human beings without a valid license. The defendant was sentenced to seven days imprisonment in jail, and ordered to pay a fine of $100 and costs. Justice Sullivan added that he could not approve of the method employed by the investigator for the State, who falsely informed the defendant as to her physical condition, thereby inducing the defendant to commit the offense charged.[11]

In the late 1940s, things started to change when the naprapathic profession, screaming for more insight—more knowledge of how the body works—took the next step forward itself. In 1948, a group of naprapathic physicians, including Dr. Fonda Stewart and her husband, Dr. Paul Stewart, Dr. Ford Roberts, Dr. Harvey Hafemeister, and his wife, Dr. Frieda Hafemeister, started their own naprapathic school, the National Naprapathic College, with a curriculum that boldly included the basic sciences. Though their own naprapathic education had been lacking in this knowledge, the group hired every expert they could lay their hands on. They were also granted a state charter to confer naprapathic degrees, but they could not coordinate efforts to apply for licensing as long as Oakley, with his strong presence and refusal to compromise to meet the state's scientific educational demands, was alive.

When Oakley died in 1957, the professional momentum of his school began to decline, ultimately leading (in 1964) to the two schools, which were Illinois not-for-profit corporations, combining as a corporate merger. They were integrated to form the Chicago National College of Naprapathy. So, the profession started small, and by 1980s, when I began my studies, was still not very large. There was one small school in Chicago and one other in Europe.

When I started school, naprapaths, students, and the college were actively contributing to a lobbyist in Springfield, Illinois's capitol, in an attempt to get the profession properly licensed. Stories would come back that although we'd paid the lobbyist to talk to the legislators, and although the legislators said they would support the bill, when the vote came up, it seemed that their urge to urinate was stronger than the commitment they had made to us. It wasn't that they voted "no," they just weren't present to vote at all—they were *accidentally* in the bathroom.

It was amazing how we poured what little money the profession had into Springfield. Naprapathy is not a large profession. We're not like the AMA, with thousands of MDs in the state, each giving money every month to pay for lobbying power. We don't have that kind of clout: clout that can run a state. Naprapathy was a little-known profession, and naprapaths eked out a living, lovingly helping patients with noninvasive, drugless healing.

Then came the revision of the Medical Practice Act, sometimes referred to as the "sunset year" in which a periodic review of government agencies, programs, or legislation is done to determine the need for revision and/or dismantling. The Illinois legislature put their heads together, with the help of the AMA's lobbyists, to rewrite the act in terms of who could be a drugless physician—the revision took out that nebulous wording "any healing system or method" and replaced it with "only chiropractors." Drugless physicians no longer included naprapaths. Suddenly it was a felony to practice naprapathy.

Originally, naprapaths had been included as legitimate health practitioners under the drugless physician portion of the act. But with the new revision, only the "big three"—medical doctors, osteopaths, and chiropractors—could touch or give medical treatments to the spine. This forced the naprapathic profession to run the gauntlet of the Illinois judicial system all the way to the state Supreme Court. But this was not our first trip. Three years prior to that we had made the expensive and time-consuming journey, with wonderful results. Finally, in 1986, the Supreme Court upheld the right of Dr. Maryann Potts to practice naprapathy, which it considered a system of treating human ailments, and that naprapaths were eligible for examination and licensure.[12] It ordered the state to begin the procedure to license naprapaths.

The second Supreme Court ruling in 1989, however, upheld the revision to the Medical Practice Act that allowed only medical doctors, chiropractors, and osteopaths to touch or medically treat the spine—allowed only these three groups to practice naprapathy—never mind the fact that they had no desire to do so.

Fortunately, some of the college's graduates during these troubled years turned out to be bright young aggressive thinkers.

The changing tide needed these dynamic new caretakers to help a profession that had been stuffed in a closet for too many years. Dr. Glenn Smith, Dr. Mide Szarmac, Dr. Robert Svast, and Dr. Rich Schaefer, who had all graduated in the mid-1980s, became members of the Illinois Naprapathic Association's board. Given the okay from the American Naprapathic Association, which consisted of the entire membership of the Chicago National College of Naprapathy, our representative approached the chiropractic profession asking for help. In response, the chiropractors graciously put together an accelerated program that would lead most of us naprapaths to a chiropractic degree. Thus, we went back to the naprapathic profession with a proposal that would grandfather in certain naprapaths who had been in practice for a certain amount of years and would implement a chiropractic program for anyone who had not been in practice long enough to be grandfathered in. An election was conducted allowing all the members of the naprapathic not-for-profit corporation, which was also the degree granting authority of the naprapathic school. The entire membership of The Chicago National College of Naprapathy ("CNCN") narrowly approved the agreement negotiated with the National College of Chiropractic ("NCC"). But those who opposed the plan began litigation against CNCN and NCC that lasted the entire time we attended chiropractic school.

So, the chiropractic-naprapathy students were forced to hire their own set of lawyers. The debate centered on whether this contract with the chiropractors was a merger—a term that had appeared on the ballot when the profession voted on whether to support the newly proposed chiropractic program. Although a lower Illinois court ruled that, indeed, this was no merger, the real hot spot of contention centered around who controlled the degree granting, not-for-profit corporation known as the Chicago National College of Naprapathy. The straight naprapaths saw the future of their profession being put on a shelf and forgotten if the chiropractors retained possession of the corporation.

The naprapathic chiropractors saw the future of the naprapathy as being null and void if compromises were not made.

Things got hot, and people became irritated. There were stories of tires being slashed. Someone broke the office windows of the woman heading the chiropractic-naprapathy faction. And the police were called to chaperone the association meetings because of intense bickering, fueled by the fact that a few of the members consumed too much alcohol. These were silly pranks committed by an angry profession split in two.

How could a profession that had been around since 1908, helping to make people healthy, be considered a felony? Young doctors struggling to start a practice and pay school debts (often working another job to support their families) were not anxious to tear their lives apart in order to retrain for another medical career. First of all, most naprapaths think the chiropractic profession is too rough and pays way too little attention to the fact that muscle, tendon, and ligaments play a major role in spinal misalignment. Why spend another $20,000 to $25,000, not to mention the loss of income for three years, to study a profession they did not want? Medical freedom! Where was it? Were we going to be forced to go to Europe or South America to practice a system of healing that gets good results, just because it did not have enough money behind its lobbying effort? Half of the profession refused to be retrained.

With legislation in place supporting the demise of the naprapathic profession, the Illinois Department of Professional Regulation traveled to Ottawa, Illinois, and went undercover to ensnare a naprapath administering calcium for muscular-skeletal problems, slapping him with 20 counts of practicing medicine without a license. This action brought the reality and the severity of our position to a clearer light for the profession. Many practicing naprapaths closed their doors, removed their shingles, and quietly took their names out of the phone book. Many only saw existing patients.

And others began to do simple massage only. From behind closed shutters, everybody waited.

Mindful of the fact that a program had been established to retrain naprapaths, the State of Illinois also waited after showing its strong presence while part of the naprapath profession finished its chiropractic education. The state was aware that the students were making progress and trying to come to terms with this new Medical Practice Act. And it waited patiently, even though this litigation in Ottawa was hanging over the naprapathic profession, threatening each and every one of us with charges of practicing medicine without a license.

Although the program set up by the chiropractic profession was a trade in money for education, the fact that the state not-for-profit naprapathic corporation was in the possession of the faction that had instituted the program, was a pivotal point. The future of naprapathy was tied to the fate of that corporation. The hierarchy within the chiropractic profession had hopes of eventually using the naprapathic degree granting aspect of the corporation to offer chiropractic physicians an advanced degree in naprapathy. Although the chiropractic graduate curriculum already included programs in radiology and acupuncture, I was certain this plan would have introduced the small naprapathic profession to the world beyond the State of Illinois. It would have taught every chiropractor who delivers those hard, fast, chiropractic thrusts that soft tissue needs more gentle massage-like manipulation for the treatment to have longer-lasting results.

We kept the lawyers on retainer until every single one of us had graduated from the chiropractic program. With our education completed, the peace talks began. The naprapathic profession would be split into two factions. Several hundred thousand dollars, the property, and the building that housed the college would be divided equally. The naprapathic chiropractors would begin repaying their sizable school loans. Meanwhile, the straight naprapaths would invest their half of the money in lobbying the state, once again, in an effort to get another law passed. This law would separate them from the medical professionals of the Medical Practice Act but allow them to practice naprapathy legally in Illinois. And damned if they didn't get just that! I guess all they needed was a lot more money.

The provisions of the bill stipulated that they were required to establish a committee comprised of naprapaths and medical doctors that would put together a comprehensive test for those graduating after 1984. The state was a little slow—no—the state was snail-like in forming the testing committee. It took three years. In November of 1997, the first test to apply for an Illinois naprapathic license was taken by 28 naprapaths. Dr. Phil Santino informed me that forty percent passed. In May of that same year, another test was offered by the State and 17 naprapaths took it, but only two passed. Time will tell the uncertain future of the naprapaths.

---

1. *Oakley Smith's Schism of 1908: The Rise and Decline of Naprapathy* By Dr. Ronald Beideman, D.C., F.I.C.C. 1994.

2. *The Connective Tissue Monograph* by Oakley Smith, 1919.

3. *Oakley Smith's Tissue Monograph, Naprapathic Connectivology* Vol. 1, 1919.

4. The Oakley Smith College of Naprapathy. *Oakley Smith's Schism of 1908: The Rise And Decline of Naprapathy* by Dr. Ronald P. Beideman, D.C., F.I.C.C. 1994.

5. People v. Lucius J. Love, 298 Ill. p. 305, 1921.

6. People v. Love.

7. Love, 298 Ill. p. 305, 1921.

8. People v. Witte, 315 Ill. 282, 146 N.E. p. 178, 1924.

9. People v. Witte, 315 Ill. 282, 146 N.E. p. 178, 1924.

10. People v. Barnes, 240 Ill. App. p. 357, 1926.

11. People v. Elmore, 17 N.E.2d p. 234, 1938.

12. Maryann Potts v. State of Illinois Department of Registration and Education, 128 Ill.2d pp. 322, 326 1986.

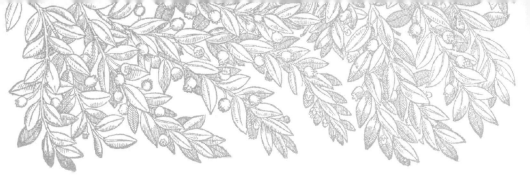

Afterword

How many chiropractors does it take to change a light bulb? Only one, but it requires 57 visits!

Of course, I strongly suggest that you avoid any healer, be it chiropractor, naprapath, or osteopath, who requires you to sign an agreement for 57 sessions. Exercise regularly and listen to your body. When it needs stretching, circulation, and the energy that can only come through a real healer's hands, go ahead and make an appointment. Take one treatment at a time, and re-book at the first sign that your condition is changing for the worse. Keep re-booking periodically, every three weeks to three months, because you will stay healthier with preventive care. I guarantee that areas of tension that you had no idea existed will make themselves known as soon as someone starts rubbing.

Try to stop the busy runaround of your life and take care of yourself. Take care of your back. Spend the money. If you're happy, and you vibrate with all the possible energy the Great Spirit has to give, you'll be able to transfer that happiness and give it to all those you take care of—whether it is your children, your spouse, or just the people in your environment. A healthy you, with respect to your body, will vibrate throughout your surroundings and be reflected back many times over. Give and you shall receive.

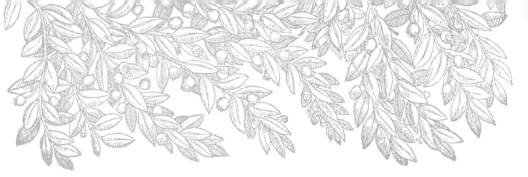

Contacts

Rio Caliente Hot Spring Spa
U.S. Address - P.O. Box 897
Millbrae, California
Phone: 650-615-9543
Fax: 650-615-0601
E-Mail: RioCal@aol.com

Sir Jason Winters
P.O. Box 94075
Las Vegas, NV 89193
E-Mail: winters04@aol.com
url: www.sirjasonwinters.com

Natural Ovens of Manitowoc
P.O. Box 730
Manitowoc, WI 54221-0730
Phone 800/772-0730

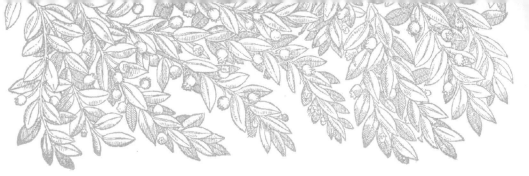

Index

A

Acid, 4

Acidic, 41

Adrenal exhaustion, 95

Algae, 122

Alkaline, 4

Alkalinizing foods, 41

Allergies, 130

Angelica pubescens, 101

Angelica sinenses, 101

Antidepressant, 125

Apple cider vinegar, 17

Arthritis, 141

Artificial sugar, 76-77

Artificial sweeteners, 92

Athlete's foot, 83

Atlas, 56

B

B-complex, 31, 66-67, 87, 89, 94, 98, 106, 116

Back-of-the-Head Headaches, 69

Bee Pollen, 119

Blue-Green Algae, 122

Breath, 112

Bronchitis, 94

Bursitis, 94

C

Caffeinated, 3

Caffeine, 8, 78, 92

Caffeine-free soda pop, 3

Calcium, 4, 70

Calcium citrate, 8

Calcium Inhibitors, 6

Cancer, 93

Cancerous, 124, 130

Carpal-Tunnel Syndrome, 66, 104

Castor oil compress, 129–32
    effect on brain   130–31

Chamomile, 103

Chiropractor, 11

Chlorella, 122

Chlorophyll, 5

Coffee, 8, 51, 76, 79, 87, 91-93, 105, 115, 142

Cold, 92

Cold water, 78

Comfrey Root, 132

Congested lung, 122

Congestion, ear and sinus 65

Constipated, 130

D

Dandelions, 121

Dark-green leafy, 89

Decaffeinated coffee, 93

Depression, 100, 104

Digestive disturbances, 92

Disc, 42, 141

Disease complex, 23

Dr. Oakley Smith "The Father of Naprapathy", 151

Dressing, 89

Drinks, 87

E

Ear congestion, 65

Echinacea, 100

Epsom salts, 17, 126

Exercises, 47–52, 108–110

F

Female cycle HA, 79–81

Female reproductive organs, 100, 130, 135

Front-of-the-Head Headaches, 76

G

Greens, 7

Gypsum, 141

H

Hay fever, 148

Headaches, 69
  Back-of-the-Head, 69-76
  Front-of-the-Head, 76-79

Healing crisis, 15

Heart, 66-67, 110, 135, 143

Heat, 36

Herbal supplements, 8

Hip rotation, 25-26, 41

Hips, 24

Homeopathic remedy, 74

Hormonal, 79-81

Hormonal headaches, 79

Hot, 126

Hot and Cold Therapy, 20-21, 31

Hot flashes, 79

Hot Packs or Cold Packs, 18

I

Ice-cold, 87

Infertility, 136

Itching, 139

J

Jason Winters Tea, 78, 91, 114

K

Kidney, 136, 142

Knees, 41, 143

L

Lower Back, 47, 143

Lungs, 136

M

Magnesium, 4

Masada, 126

Masada bath salts, 17

Menopause, 79

Menstrual pain, 9

Mineral springs, 17

Mineral water, 126

Muscle spasms, 21

Muscular spasms, 3

N

Naprapath, xii, 11

Naprapathy, xii, 150

Neck, 55

Neck-traction, 65

Nerve, 98

Nerves, 85

No. 1 cream, 141

No. 2 cream, 139

Numbness, 66, 86, 105

Nutri-Stars, 89

O

Osteoporosis, 1, 5

Oyster shells, 8

P

Painful elbow, 66

Panax ginseng, 101

Phosphorous, 4, 77

PMS, 79-80, 135

Protective muscle spasm, 23

Psoriasis, 139

R

Rashes, 139

Reflexology, 40

Rescue Remedy, 74-76, 80

Rio Caliente, 126

Root canal, 131

Rotation, 24

Rubefacient, 19

S

Salts, 126

Saliva militiorrhiza, 101

Sciatic nerve, 28–30, 8–86, 90

Sciatica, 28, 30

Sinus congestion, 92

Sources of Calcium, 6

Spinus process, 12

Spirulina, 122

Stomach, 80, 92, 136, 138

Sugar, 90, 98, 116

T

Tea Tree Oil, 132

Teeth, 143

Tension, 57

Tension headaches, 73

The Third-World Squat, 49

Thinning hair, 142

Thoracic Outlet Syndromes, 104

Transverse process, 56

U

Uterus, 136

V

Vertebra, 12

Vitamin B-Complex, 85

Vitamins, 7

W

Water-soluble, 7

White-flour bread, 90, 105

Women's Precious, 79

Y

Yang, 96

Yin, 96

Z

Zheng Gu Shui, 18, 76, 133, 141

Dr. Schmidt's Pharmacopoeia

Price List

Dr. Schmidt's Herbal Calcium Minerals		$12.00
#1 Chinese Cream	small	$7.00
#1 Chinese Cream	large	$22.00
#2 Chinese Cream	small	$7.00
#2 Chinese Cream	large	$22.00
Women's Precious		$17.00
Circulation Formula		$17.00
Zheng Gu Shui Liniment Spray		$10.00
Jason Winters Tea		$8.00
B-Complex Complete		$28.00

Orders payable by check, Visa, Mastercard, or Discover. If paying by check, please include $2.50 S/H for 1–3 items or $3.50 S/H for 4-6 items. Illinois residents should also include 7.75% sales tax.

If ordering from outside the Continental U.S., call for shipping rates.

Phone, Fax, Mail or E-mail your order with payment to:

Dr. Marcia Schmidt
509 West Main Street
Barrington, IL 60010

Phone: 847/381-8459
Fax: 847/277-0214
E-mail: dr_marcia_schmidt@ameritech.net

Or order from her website at: www.prcinc.net/dr_schmidt.htm